THE CALORIE FALLACY

THE CALORIE FALLACY

weigh less by eating more

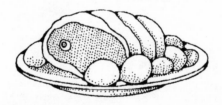

Barry A Groves

BOOKMARQUE

PUBLISHERS & TYPESETTERS

Minster Lovell & New Yatt · Oxfordshire

A BOOKMARQUE GENERAL
Published by Bookmarque Publishing
Minster Lovell & New Yatt · Oxfordshire

First published 1994
Reprinted September 1997

© Barry A Groves 1997

ISBN 1-870519–29–9

British Library Cataloguing in Publication Data
A catalogue record for this book is available from the British Library

---

Edited by T C Colverson
Printed by Antony Rowe Ltd

CONTENTS

ACKNOWLEDGEMENTS

I must thank all the people without whose help I could not have written this book. Firstly, Dr Richard Mackarness, whose book *Eat Fat and Grow Slim* changed my life so radically for the better over thirty years ago. Next my wife, Monica, who has spent many hours in stuffy libraries helping me to search the medical journals; and for her tolerance when the garden has come a poor second to my writing. Lastly, all my friends who have put up with me, read the book at various stages and helped with their suggestions.

Barry A Groves

May 1994

My sincere thanks to all those who kindly bought a copy of the first edition of my book which has, more by word of mouth than anything else, generated enough continuing demand to necessitate this reprint.

Barry A Groves

September 1997

One must attend in medical practice not primarily to plausible theories but to experience combined with reason. Hippocrates

INTRODUCTION

Walk into any large newsagent's shop today and count the number of slimming magazines. Then add the number of slimming articles in women's magazines. Now ask yourself why there are so many. The answer is: they don't work! These publications are in business to make a profit, to increase their market share and, primarily, to stay in business. If they published a diet which really did slim people as easily and permanently as they all say they will, no-one would need to buy the next edition. They would be committing commercial suicide.

Present dietary regimes
Over the past twenty or more years a number of diet books and regimes have been marketed with miraculous claims for their effects. They all claim that a dieter can lose more weight than is safe, yet be safe. One has only to read the medical journals to discover how untrue that statement is. These diets tend to have three things in common: they all restrict fats, they all restrict calories and they all don't work. You might lose some weight but in over 90% of cases it soon goes on again. So you try another diet, buy another book or join another club – and spend some more money.

Make no mistake, slimming is a multi-million-pound business. Over 90% of the British population has tried dieting at some time or other, and at any one time a third of the adult population is trying to lose weight. In Britain alone, we spend £850 million a year on it and a prosperous slimming industry can look forward with confidence to a never-ending income as articles that promise unattainable goals persuade women (mostly) to attempt the impossible. The magazines know that many women are so desperate to lose weight that, although they constantly fail, they will try any and every new diet that comes

9

along. Whatever it is, they want to be the first to try it. It is not a new phenomenon; as long ago as 29 March 1957, a 17-stone woman appeared on the ITV programme *State Your Case for £100*. She said that she wanted the money so that she could attend what she called a 'slimming farm'. She did not get the money. No doubt if she had had £100 at the time she would have spent it all on slimming. The fact that she appeared on the programme in front of millions of viewers demonstrated the strength of her need. So the magazines publish diet after diet – all destined to fail. But fail in such a way that they make women need the next one. It's an addiction. And an addiction which is created and nurtured by the slimming and food industries. For example, did you know that Weight-Watchers, probably the best known slimming organisation, is a wholly owned subsidiary of Heinz Foods?

So, what should you be eating to reduce to and maintain a normal weight? There are so many apparently conflicting theories about diet. Weight control combined with good nutrition need be neither dreary nor difficult. *The Calorie Fallacy* looks at our evolution to see what foods we are adapted to eat. It discusses the reasons we, as a species, get fat, and it explores the history of slimming over the past 130 years. It also contains yet another dietary regime. It may seem a revolutionary regime but it is not a new one, merely out of fashion. It is one which is both natural and healthy but, more than that, it is easy to follow. Unlike all the others around today, it has been proven to work in medical trials conducted over half a century. This should come as no surprise as *The Calorie Fallacy* presents a regime which is a natural diet for our species.

The Calorie Fallacy really began in 1962 when I was working in Singapore as an electronic engineer with the Royal Air Force. We had a problem, my wife and I – we were very overweight.

We had tried all the usual ways to lose weight: cutting calories, eating inert fillers, taking appetite suppressants. Unfortunately, the results were decidedly short-term and unprofitable. And then the first moment of revelation came, sudden and unexpected, when I was walking through the bustling Changi Market in Singapore. I saw a second-hand bookstall and, as I am an inveterate browser, stopped to see what was on offer. One small paperback stood out. That book changed our lives – and our figures – for good.

The book advocated what we thought was impossible: a high-calorie diet for weight loss. It said in so many words: Eat as many calories as you like, and the pounds will fall away. Because this proposition seemed so out of keeping with all we had read up to that time, we decided to see what it could do for us. To our astonishment, it worked, and it has gone on working for over thirty years.

Then the questions began: If an unlimited-calorie diet can achieve such results, why are all the books and magazine articles in favour of calorie-controlled diets? I began my research and the answers came. All the evidence I found persuaded me that low-calorie dieting is a snare for the overweight and a delusion for all concerned.

Later we began to hear that the diet we had been following, relatively high in animal fats, might be dangerous in terms of increased risk of coronary heart disease.

And so, when I retired from the Royal Air Force in 1982, and had time enough, I devoted myself to a full-time literature search into the healthiness of 'healthy eating'. I began in the medical library of a major teaching hospital; and I chased after the more recondite topics in Oxford's Bodleian and Radcliffe Science Libraries. All too soon I found that, contrary to what we read in so many books and articles, there was little evidence to show that 'healthy eating' is good for the health or the figure.

As I read on and on, it dawned on me that a vast 'health' industry did a very good business of offering expensive solutions for the problems, so they said, of keeping ourselves slim and fit. All those adverts on television – eat this, try that diet – could they have anything to do with the profit motive?

Cholesterol, saturated fat, the more you eat, the more likely you are to end up with Heart Disease. Cut down on calories; eat specially prepared, nutritionally-poor but very expensive 'healthy' or 'slimming' foods. There is no doubt that the food industry was very quick to see the profits that could be made out of frightening people. Others too saw their chance and climbed on the bandwagon. Slimming magazines and clubs sprang up almost overnight. Vast sums are invested in making people feel dissatisfied with themselves so the they will spend even larger sums trying to change.

Belief versus truth

Once upon a time, our ancestors believed in many things which we know today are untrue: that the world was flat; that men could be changed into toads; that the lungs were a furnace in which fats and carbohydrates were burned to warm the body. Today, anyone who professed such beliefs would be described as 'old-fashioned' or 'crassly ignorant'. We believe that we have replaced such superstitions with proven scientific facts. But have we? How do we know that the beliefs we hold true today are not destined to become the superstitions of tomorrow? If history teaches us anything, it is that many certainly will be.

Science has always progressed by demolishing established beliefs. Every time it makes a breakthrough, it marks the demise of some previously accepted conclusion. For this reason, we should always be tentative in our beliefs. At one time, it was believed that the Earth was the centre of the universe; that the Sun, planets and stars all revolved around it. So strong and so universal was the belief that anyone who doubted it and expressed those doubts was labelled a heretic and, in many cases, put to death.

Intensity of conviction, however, is no guarantee of truth. To know the truth of our beliefs, we must test them and prove them, and to do this we must use reason. Many truths we hold, of course, are proven already. For example, we know that 2+2=4 and that the moon goes round the Earth and the Earth round the Sun. We take these beliefs on trust: they were hypothesised by scientists long ago, and have been checked and re-checked many times since to prove their veracity.

So beliefs change. The ones that remain are those that can be proven to be true. We should not cling to disproven beliefs out of a sense of loyalty and a faith in the familiar. In things scientific we should keep an open mind. If a belief is shown to be untrue, it should be discarded.

At one time there was a philosophical maxim that 'all clear ideas are true'. It is demonstrably unsound, but no maxim conforms more exactly to human nature. Unless we are careful, the mere presentation of an idea makes us believe it, and if others believe it also, that quickly adds to our belief.

The ease with which our minds accept certain ideas as true is one of the greatest barriers to clear thinking. We must break down this barrier by recognising this weakness: by realising that our minds, like our bodies, are slaves to habit. In childhood, we have a voracious appetite for knowledge and an immense curiosity. A child will accept everything it is told as true. At that stage, we have yet to develop the power of weighing the evidence. We have no concept of ideas which are merely unproven hypotheses or which are false. In consequence, we accept everything as true and go on believing it until such time as bitter experience proves it to be false. Sometimes, even then we go on believing it. But in childhood, we not only acquire beliefs, we also acquire attitudes of mind, prejudices, enthusiasms, fears and hopes which we cling to usually throughout life.

It is much easier to instil a new idea into a person's head than it is to eradicate or modify an old one. Thus people have great difficulty in discarding the idea that low-calorie dieting does not work, as it has been the perceived wisdom for generations. Most people also like to be the same and say the same as their peers: they do not like being thought of as unusual. They will go along with something because 'everybody says so'. And the more people say something, the more it will be believed – whether it is true or not.

The power of suggestion

Many of our beliefs are not held because we have verified them for ourselves but for other reasons ranging from the influence of what we are taught in childhood to what we see on television or read in the newspapers. Although these influences have different origins, they all have one factor in common. That is their appeal to and effect upon our suggestibility. We humans are immensely responsive to suggestion – a fact that is used with great success by the advertising companies.

Most people will accept as true any statement which is expressed clearly, simply and confidently. Its effect is greatly enhanced if it is repeated often. For example, if a friend remarked to you: 'Smith's low-fat jam is good for you', you would probably note it but put it out of your mind and forget it. If, however, you saw 'BUY SMITH'S LOW-FAT JAM', in shops, newspapers and on television, you would probably buy it. If it is sold with an appeal to its prestige value or promoted as being healthy, you are even more likely to buy it.

Many worthless things, including ideas, can be sold in this way. You might suppose that the value of the merchandise or idea would exercise a check on the power of advertising; that once it is found to be false or worthless, that would be the end of it. It is a sad fact, however, that very few people profit from experience. Despite having been fooled in the past, low-calorie slimmers still allow themselves to be deceived again and again with successive low-calorie diets and pay heavily for their gullibility. In these times, scepticism is a trait to be nurtured. You must learn not to accept hypotheses as true until they have been tested and can be shown to be true.

The Calorie Fallacy questions the perceived wisdom of low-calorie slimming diets because they have never been tested and shown to work. It questions them because history and numerous scientifically conducted clinical trials have shown that their whole philosophy is wrong.

Fats and health

This book advocates a diet which is relatively high in fat. Back in the 1950s this would not have been thought odd. However, dietary fat has had such a bad press recently that to advocate today a diet which is high in fat, could make the average dietitian shudder. But in the medical journals a great debate rages and, like all debates, it has two sides. Slimming and health are big business. Without fat people, the slimming industry would crumble, without ill-health we would not need a health service. They all have vested interests. As a consequence, they have subjected you to only one side of the debate. One thing I can promise: A rare opportunity to hear the other side of the slimming and health arguments and the evidence on which they are based. *The Calorie Fallacy* presents the evidence that the experts have presented. The final judgement rests with you. The father of medicine, Hippocrates, wrote: 'One must attend in medical practice not primarily to plausible theories but to experience combined with reason'. This is the attitude to adopt when considering which dietary regime is most likely to be healthy.

The end of the 20th century has seen a proliferation of dietary myths and fads. For the most part they are fraudulent, designed to relieve as many people of as much money as they can. Low-calorie dieting is a major fraud. In the 19th century William Banting wrote of a slimming diet which worked. In the 20th century it was tested extensively. By the 21st century, with the frauds exposed, that vile word 'obese' could become obsolete and disappear from our language for good.

Fashion, though Folly's child, and guide of fools,
Rules e'en the wisest, and in learning rules.
George Crabbe.

1
IS YOUR DIET REALLY NECESSARY?

You probably would not have bought this book if you did not believe that you were at least slightly overweight. Models on catwalks, pictures in fashion magazines, and the slimming industry may have convinced you that you should shed a few pounds. But are you sure that you are overweight? It is important, as you should never try to lose weight if you are not overweight.

There is no doubt that to be too much overweight is not a desirable state, at least from a medical standpoint. Being obese is generally not socially acceptable, but more than this, being excessively overweight puts unnecessary strains on the heart, and back and knee joints. It also makes any surgery more difficult. But are you really overweight? Fads come and go, fashions change, how can you tell?

There are a number of ways to measure whether you are the right weight for your height: skin-fold thickness, body density measurement, height/weight tables, and so on. Height/weight tables are the criteria that most people use, so, in this book, we will concentrate on those. The generally recognised definition of overweight is a weight which is above the acceptable weight for your height, and obesity is defined as being 20% or more above the upper limit of the acceptable weight range. Having said that, however, we have to define 'acceptable' as there are now known to be health risks associated with extreme leanness – it is safer to be overweight than underweight.

The acceptable weight ranges at present are those shown in Appendix A. In these tables, however, women's acceptable weights range considerably lower than those for men, and, as there is no reason why they should, weights of the two sexes are currently being brought into line. You will also notice that the small/medium/large frame sizes have disappeared. This is because these were always artificial; doctors had asked for them and the acceptable ranges were split arbitrarily into three. There is no scientific definition of frame size.

The weight ranges for any particular height may seem very wide as they cover a band of nearly 30 lbs for a woman of 4 ft 9 ins to over 40 lbs for a tall man, but there is no evidence that weight at one position within this range is any healthier than at any other position. A weight at the top is as healthy as one in the middle or one at the bottom. A person's weight wanders about constantly over a few pounds and many people worry quite unnecessarily about their weights.

Unfortunately, the old tables are still being used in current diet books and slimming magazines; the concept of frame sizes, for example, was abandoned as long ago as 1973. But slimming is a multi-million-pound industry. If people are told that they ought not to be so thin after all, the industry could lose some of its business – and that is not their aim. And as muscle is heavier than fat, a body builder with no excess body fat can weigh the same as a person of similar height with considerably more body fat.

Other tests whereby you pinch a fold of flesh on the upper arm to gauge the amount of fat are more realistic as they are more individual. But a figure of three-quarters of an inch, generally regarded as the norm, does not allow for individual physiology. Another good way to test whether you are overweight is to look at your face. If it is neither bloated around the eyes, which would be an indication of overweight, nor hollowed, an indication of underweight, you are at your ideal weight. If you do not feel you are overweight, then you are probably not.

Fashions Change
In primitive societies it is often fatness which is desired; in the West it is more likely to be slimness. Slimming magazines, women's fashions and the media portray the desirable woman as tall and thin. We live in a time when slimness is the fashion but it was not always so – fashions change. Centuries ago celibate early Christian writers were terrified of women's flesh. They were frightened by their own lascivious thoughts – but put the blame on women. In an attempt to make women as sexless as possible, the Church urged women to fast. Travel through time to the 16th and 17th centuries and the fashion had changed dramatically. Rubens' paintings depict women who are considerably more cuddly. At the beginning of the 20th century it was also fashionable to be buxom. By the 1920s, however, busts were out and it was fashionable to be slim once more. In the 1930s the fashion changed to cuddly again – and back

yet again with Twiggy in the 1960s. The Twiggy look has persisted.

However, we should be less concerned with what is fashionable and concentrate more on what is normal and what is healthy. In reality, the women employed in the fashion business today are not normal, they are freaks. The only safe way to look like them is to be born like them. But why would any woman want to look like them? Ask most men, for example, what shape they desire in a woman, and you will find that they prefer one considerably more rounded. Indeed the major difference between the sexes is that healthy men tend to be hard and angular and healthy women soft and rounded. To know what shape a man prefers, look at the centrefold of a man's magazine. The ideal shape, from both a desirability and a health point of view, is nearer to that seen in paintings by Rubens than on the cat-walk.

In both sexes, body fat plays an important role. It fills hollows in the skeleton, the eye sockets, joints and neck. It cushions and protects internal organs and provides a reservoir of energy. It is fat which contours the body: when the body loses fat, it sags and shows the signs of ageing. Body fat is synonymous with the looks and actions of youth.

Women have more fat cells than men. In a woman, up to 24% of body weight should be fat; in men only about 12% should be fat. Curves distinguish women from men. The woman's extra fat is both a natural and a normal phenomenon brought about by the sex hormones during puberty. As well as having an aesthetic value, it is of biological importance, preparing the woman for motherhood. A feminine body is a curvaceous body. Why try to lose it? It is much the healthier attitude to be satisfied with what you have rather than continually try to change it.

The dangers of low-calorie slimming

However, if you must lose weight, check with your doctor to ensure that it is necessary. This is particularly important if you are only mildly or moderately overweight and thinking of embarking on a 'crash' diet, as you are at increased risk of arrhythmic sudden death on such diets. And diet in a way that is safe. There is a serious risk of harm on very-low-calorie liquid-protein diets such as the Cambridge Diet even under medical supervision. The 'yo-yo' effect of rapid weight loss, followed inevitably by weight gain, repeated over and over is far more dangerous to health than a high but steady weight.

Gallstone formation is usually thought of as a result of being too heavy but drastic very low calorie dieting is much more likely to be the cause. Most diets restrict fats. But when a low-fat diet is eaten, the gall bladder, which stores the bile, is not emptied. This means that bile remains relatively stagnant allowing gallstones to form. In a study of gallstone formation, conducted in America in 1989, obese patients were put on a 500-calorie-a-day high-protein, low-fat diet. Those taking part were very carefully screened at the start of the study to ensure that none had any sign of gallbladder disease, but during only eight weeks, 25% of the subjects developed gallstones. This is an alarming finding as gallstones are not only painful, the operation to remove them is potentially life-threatening. The more one uses low-fat diets, the greater is the risk.

Slimming, therefore, is a serious and risky business which should not be embarked upon lightly. How many slimming magazines explain this to their readers? They all give the impression that losing weight is always beneficial.

Slimming clubs and counsellors are only too aware that the modern slimmer will sacrifice anything to lose weight. They set unreasonably low target weights and encourage unreasonably rapid weight loss. Many slimmers find these regimes impossible to resist. Do they work? Yes, but only in the short term, and then the weight returns. After losing 140 lbs in a year and becoming the 1980 Weight Watcher of the Year, the recipient of this honour said that the experience had changed his life. Suddenly, he was no longer a loser but a success. But the euphoria did not last for long. As soon as he had reached his target weight, the weight he had lost began to return. After a 12-year struggle, his weight in 1992 was 21 stones – right back where it started. Interviewed on television, he said that the whole weight-loss philosophy was wrong. Slimmers' minds are focused and concentrated on food, when food is the last thing they should be thinking about. He went on to say that his mood now was one of depression, disappointment and a loss of self-esteem; feelings all too common in the long-term slimmer.

There are many people who are not even slightly overweight, much less obese, who have been started by all the publicity on an unnecessary slimming programme which will ultimately have an adverse effect on their bodies' regulatory systems. Unfortunately, adolescent girls seem to have an exaggerated concern about getting fat regardless of whether they are overweight or not. A recently published study even shows that as many as 51% of those who were *underweight* expressed extreme anxiety about being overweight and over a third were preoccupied with body fat. In a society obsessed with body weight, even young girls who are underweight are dieting. Such inappropriate eating patterns are associated with many medical problems and poor growth.

Parents who are dieting also tend to put their young offspring on similar low-calorie diets. This can have devastating results. A growing child needs lots of protein to build body tissue. As a child's stomach is relatively small, he or she must have a diet which contains lots of energy. Low-fat, low-calorie slimming diets should have no place in the life of anyone prior to puberty.

You should never try to lose weight if you are not overweight. If you are at your correct weight and maintain it without dieting, you have no need to diet. Having said that, however, this book may still be of interest as, if the principles of the dietary regime detailed are followed, you will not become overweight.

> **The first rule is:**
> **If you are not overweight, don't diet.**

We must, however, acknowledge . . . that man with all his noble qualities, still bears in his bodily frame the indelible stamp of his lowly origin. Charles Darwin.

2
CARBOHYDRATE - THE REAL CULPRIT

Over the last decade, we have been told incessantly to reduce our intake of fat. But we cannot merely eat less of a major part of our diet without making up the deficit with something else. Containing as it does over 9 calories per gram, fat is the best provider of energy. Cut out fat and you need to eat more than twice as much protein or carbohydrate to make up the shortfall. Whether from meat or vegetable sources such as nuts, foods high in proteins also tend to be relatively high in fat. This leaves those who would change us to a 'healthier' lifestyle with no other option but to recommend that we increase our intake of foods which are rich in carbohydrates.

During the history of mankind and particularly in this century, many studies have been carried out into the role that the various foodstuffs play in the aetiology of diseases. Fats and proteins have always been classed as beneficial. Indeed, in the 1950s fat was called 'the most valuable food known to man'. It was not until the seemingly inexorable rise in heart disease in the middle of the twentieth century which had to be explained, that fat started to be blamed for any disease. However, studies carried out since then, which are reviewed in Chapter Six, have shown that fats are not to blame after all.

Two types of disease
Diseases today can be split into two distinct types: diseases that are caused by living organisms such as germs and viruses, and those which are environmental. The former tend to be contagious and include such diseases as typhoid, measles and colds. The latter are ailments such as overweight, diabetes and heart disease, which are not contagious. Both have different aetiologies and both should be treated in different ways. The infectious diseases are generally

20

treated most successfully by using drugs to kill off the disease organisms. Treatment of the environmental diseases, using drugs, however, is rarely successful. Here it is better to find and modify the cause. And the cause in most cases seems to be related to the unnaturalness of our diet – no, not the fats, which usually get the blame, but the unnatural carbohydrates in our diet.

The ideal diet

Open a book by this nutritionist or that dietitian and you are likely to find contradictory views expressed. The age of the document will often reflect the current fad and, at any one time, opinions may differ. As they cannot all be right, how are we to determine what is our ideal diet?

The answer to that question lies in our past. But not the immediate past. The way we live now is based on advanced agriculture and the domestication of plants and animals. This is a very recent invention: we cannot have adapted to it yet. To determine what foods are likely to make up an ideal diet for us as a species, we must look further back, at our evolutionary history. For the food we have adapted to and should eat now is not a matter for current dietary fads, it is determined by what we have adapted to over millions of years and is coded in our genes.

We can trace Man's evolution from remains found in Africa and other parts of the world of early hominids dated as long ago as 5.5 million years. We have fossilised bone records of both man and animals. We have found stone tools and implements that must have been used for killing and cutting flesh or for grinding plants. We have even found human faeces. These findings have led to a great deal of speculation. Are we a carnivorous, omnivorous or a herbivorous species?

We call our ancestors and the various modern primitive tribes, 'hunter-gatherers'. In the world today, some tribes live exclusively on meat and fish. Others live largely on fruit, nuts and roots, although meat is also highly prized. It is obvious, therefore, that we can survive on a wide variety of foods. But which, if any, is ideal?

There are three possible combinations of diet we can consider: that we were wholly carnivorous, hunting and killing animals; or that we were omnivorous, eating a mixed diet of both animal and plant origin; or that we were herbivorous, i.e. vegetarians.

The vegetarian hypothesis has it that we were wholly dependent on plant foods and that meat never played an important part in our evolution. It is a hypothesis that has had fervent support in the USA.

In our hunt for an answer, the first evidence to consider lies in the fossil sites. Where hominid remains are found, so also are animal bones – at times in their thousands. If we were not meat-eaters, why is that? Secondly, although modern hunting tribes do eat plants, they have fire. Without it, there are very few plant foods with sufficient calorific value that we could have digested. There were fruits, of course, but there is not one prehistoric site in all Africa that indicates forests extensive enough to have supplied sufficient fruit to meet the needs of its inhabitants. Indeed, there is agreement that our ancestors did not dwell in forests at all but on the savannah where there were vast plains of grass. However, grass is of no value whatsoever to our digestive system. Even to live off the fleshier leaves would require the much more highly specialised digestive systems found in other primates.

Studies conducted on monkeys have led to the suggestion that the seeds of the grass could have supplied us with the energy we required. However, if this were the case, why is it that we cannot eat them now without cooking them first? Seeds, the staples such as rice, wheat, maize and beans, play an important part in our lives today. All of them, however, must be cooked before we can eat them in any quantity. Seeds and berries are a plant's reproductive system. Many are designed to attract animals and birds to eat them but there would be little point in this if the seeds were digested. No, they are indigestible – deliberately, designed to pass through the animal to be defecated and take root elsewhere. Two means only are available to make them digestible: cooking and grinding.

Before fire was harnessed, the only means by which the seeds could have been rendered digestible would have been by pounding them and breaking down the plant cell walls, but no archaeologist has ever found a Stone Age tool for this task. If chewing was the method used to do the job, a very large proportion of the seeds would escape and, passing through the body undigested, end up in the faeces. Human faeces, or coprolites as they are called, have been found and studied in detail. Older coprolites from Africa contain no plant material whatsoever. Relatively recent ones from north America have included just about everything that could remotely be called edible: from eggshells and feathers to seeds and vegetable fibres. They did eat plants – but only after they had mastered fire, and even then, many seeds had passed through undigested and unharmed. There is no doubt that the seeds cannot have been a natural part of their diet.

Homo erectus began to appreciate the value of fire around 350,000 years ago. It is true that if our ancestors had started cooking grain then, we could have evolved and adapted to it by now. However, cooking grain is not as easy as cooking meat. You cannot hang it in a chunk over the fire or lay it in the embers. To cook grain and other seeds, you need a container of some sort. The oldest known pot is only 6,800 years old. In evolutionary terms, that was only yesterday.

For any reliance on cooking, you also need a controlled fire. Although hearths have been discovered that are 100,000 years old, these are relatively rare. European Neanderthal coprolites from around 50,000 years ago, before their use of fire, contain no plant material whatsoever. It was not until Cro-Magnon's colonisation of Europe, some 35,000 years ago, that hearths became universal. However, even then they were used merely for warmth, not for cooking plants. At the time, Europe was in the grip of a succession of ice-ages. For some 70,000 years there were long, cold winters and short, cool summers. Cro-Magnon and his Eurasian ancestors cannot have been plant eaters – for most of the year there weren't any plants! He ate meat or he died. And he ate that meat raw.

The evidence was already overwhelming that we could not be a vegetarian species. However, in 1972 the publication of two independent investigations really nailed the lid on the vegetarian hypothesis' coffin. They concerned fats.

About half our brain and nervous system is composed of complicated, long-chain, fatty acid molecules. The walls of our blood vessels also need them. Without them we cannot develop normally. These fatty acids do not occur in plants. Fatty acids in a simpler form do but they must be converted into the long-chain molecules by animals – which is a slow, time-consuming process. This is where the the plant-eating herbivores come in. Over the year, they convert the simple fatty acids found in grasses and seeds into intermediate, more complicated forms. These are still not the long, complex chains that we need, but this is where the carnivores and we come in. They and we can convert the herbivore's store of the less complex fatty acids into the ones we need.

Our brain is considerably larger than that of any ape. Looking back at the fossil record from early hominids to modern man, we see a quite remarkable increase in brain size. This expansion needed large quantities of the right kinds of fatty acids before it could have occurred. It would never have occurred if our ancestors had not eaten meat. Human milk contains the fatty acids needed for large brain development – cow's milk does not. It is no coincidence that in relative terms, our brain is some fifty times the size of a cow's.

The vegetarian will be dismayed to learn that while soyabean is rich in complete protein, and grains and nuts also combine to provide complete proteins, none contains the fats that are essential for proper brain development. There is no doubt whatsoever that we cannot be a vegetarian species. From the time of *Homo erectus* some 500,000 years ago, we have lived on and adapted to a diet composed almost exclusively of meat.

All this evidence points to our being pure carnivores, as are the big cats. However, we are a remarkably successful species. It is unlikely that we would have been quite so successful if we had been forced to rely on only one source of food. It is obvious from archaeological remains that we tended when necessary to be more opportunist eaters. We hunted and ate meat primarily but, if meat was in short supply, we would eat almost anything – so long as it did not require cooking. This still precluded some of the roots and all the seeds we eat today. When meat was in short supply, we got our protein from nuts and ate fruits and berries. During our evolution, therefore, when we lived well, our diet was high in animal protein and fat: only during lean times did it include foods of vegetable origin.

So, our ideal diet, the one we evolved and adapted to, must be one which is high in proteins and fats, and low in carbohydrates.

The diet revolutions

About 9,000 years ago our ancestors started to domesticate wild grasses. From these we get the cereals we know today: wheat, barley, maize, rice, etc. We could not eat them directly as the starch molecule is too large for our digestive process to cope with. It had to be broken down first by cooking. This development began a dramatic change in Man's lifestyle. Once our ancestors produced controlled quantities of higher-energy starches which could be stored, his numbers could grow. And as numbers grew, it became more difficult to maintain his supplies through hunting. Thus his basic diet changed from a high protein/fat diet to one largely of carbohydrate.

This radical change of diet brought with it radical changes to our ancestors, both in physique and in health. As intakes of meat declined and vegetable foods made up an increasing proportion of our diet, so our height also declined. European, meat-eating *Homo erectus erectus* of 30,000 years ago was 150 mm (6 inches) taller than his agricultural descendants. Indeed, even today we are still shorter than they were. We see the same pattern in North America. The Paleoindian hunters of 10,000 years ago were much taller than their farming descendants at the time of European conquests of the 15th century AD. There is no evidence of nutritional diseases before the invention of agriculture. After it, there is. The cereal crops that became the modern staples, together with root crops which began to be cultivated, are all relatively deficient in protein and the B vitamins. Additionally, all the cereals contain a substance called phytate which binds with a number of minerals and other nutrients, and reduces their availability to the digestion. As a consequence, with the coming of agriculture we see the appearance of a number of nutritional diseases such as rickets, pellagra, dental caries, beriberi, obesity, allergies and cancers. We see the emergence of the 'diseases of civilisation'.

About 200 years ago there began a second dietary revolution which was brought about with the introduction of industrialisation. This had two powerful but opposite effects on our health. The industrialised countries, with their increased wealth, no longer had to rely on home-produced food with its seasonal changes, they could import it. Thus the populations of those countries could look forward to going through life without ever being hungry. A good thing, you might think, but it brought with it adverse effects.

Many of the imported foods were unnatural to those eating them. New fruits tasted nice and, as a consequence, we changed from eating what we needed to eating what we liked. And with no previous experience, we had never learned when to stop. At the same time, science made possible the production of synthetic foods which had the appearance, texture and taste of the real thing, but with none of the proteins and vitamins. Sugar became easy and cheap to produce, leading to a 30-fold increase in its consumption. The industrial revolution, therefore, was something of a two-edged sword. On the one hand it gave people a wider range of nutritious food than had ever before been possible; on the other it brought diabetes, peptic ulcers, heart disease and yet more dental caries, cancers and obesity.

In the late twentieth century the speed at which our diet has become increasingly unnatural has quickened. When a music hall singer at the beginning of the twentieth century sang that 'a little of what you fancy does you good', there was still an element of truth in it – at least as far as diet was concerned. When hunger signalled that the body needed more nourishment, appetite determined which elements. At one time, we ate what we had an appetite for, and the body's needs were met. Nature told us what to eat and by this means, nature ensured that we ate a balanced diet. Over the last two centuries, and increasingly during the last two decades, however, that situation has changed dramatically.

During the millions of years that we have been evolving, we have been eating natural food – our ideal diet. We had a sense of taste that told us what was good for us and what was poisonous. Like all animals on this planet, we ate what we liked without danger either from nutritional deficiency or from over-indulgence. But when food is changed from its natural state, that no longer holds true.

At first, all our food, whether from animal or vegetable sources, was eaten raw. Now cooking food has become a way of life. Most people in Western society today would not eat uncooked meat. Indeed, as possible pathogens would not be killed, it may be unwise to eat raw meat. But, while boiling parallels the first stages of digestion, and may be helpful in that process, over-cooking in a way that chars food can present the digestive processes with food which it has great difficulty digesting. In 1838 a remarkable series of experiments was performed in Canada on a man named Alexis St Martin by a Dr Beaumont. St Martin had an opening in the front wall of his stomach from a gunshot wound. Even after the wound had healed, there remained a small opening through which the mucous membrane of his stomach could be seen, and through which substances could be introduced into the stomach, or removed from it. Dr Beaumont was able to introduce foodstuffs through the opening and observe the rate of digestion. By so doing, he found that raw beef digested in 2 hours, well done boiled beef in 3 hours and well done roast beef took 4 hours. Similarly, raw eggs were digested in $1\frac{1}{2}$ hours but hard-boiled eggs took $3\frac{1}{2}$ hours.

In contrast, the cellulose which envelops cereal grains and which is the major constituent of vegetable cell walls, cannot be broken down by the digestive juices. These walls are ruptured only by the process of cooking. Cooking is also the only means of breaking down the large starch molecules so that we can digest them. As a consequence, cereals and many other vegetables need not only to be cooked, they must be well cooked, before they can be digested.

That is not to say, however, that cooking presents no problems. Cooked food, for example, can be damaging to the teeth. We know that sugar is the greatest cause of cavities in teeth, particularly children's teeth. We also know that the effect is worse if the sugary food is sticky. Dates and toffee are both high in sugars and stick around the teeth. Both, therefore, might be expected to cause cavities. But while toffee does cause dental cavities, Arabs who eat sticky, sweet dates have healthy teeth. Why the difference?

All living organism have immune systems which protect them from invading bacteria. At the time of being eaten, the raw dates are still living organisms and their immune systems are working. The bacteria which would ferment the sugars in the dates and form the acid which attacks teeth, are repelled. That is not the case with cooked and, therefore, dead toffee.

Cooking can also destroy some nutrients: Vitamin C is a good example. Thus nutrients which might be present when food is 'natural' are lost and their correct balance may also be lost.

Cooking food, therefore, may cause changes to which the body's systems are not entirely adapted and which, as a consequence may cause us minor problems. Today, however, food has been changed much more radically and in a shorter time span – a time span much too short for us to have evolved and adapted to it. A large proportion of the food we eat now can no longer be called natural. This is particularly so in the case of carbohydrates. It is this change which seems to be the cause of so many of today's ills.

There are a number of vegetable-based foods which are processed to such a high degree that nothing but pure carbohydrate is left. The obvious example is white, granulated sugar. Sugar cane and sugar beet contain a significant proportion of protein which is lost during processing. Also lost are other nutrients such as vitamins and fibre. The end product is pure, concentrated carbohydrate.

It is this concentration that is so unnatural. This has not happened with protein as it is relatively expensive. Neither has it happened with fats as they are concentrated naturally. The concentration of carbohydrate allowed a dramatic and rapid increase in its consumption. Annual sugar consumption in Britain in the middle of the eighteenth century was less than 2 kg per person, today it is more than 60 kg.

The same is true of cereals, albeit to a lesser degree. Many packaged foods today contain what is euphemistically called 'modified starch'. This again is highly concentrated carbohydrate, in this case cereal starch. This concentration of sugars and starches is done to make foods cheaper, more attractive, or to make more of a profit for the manufacturers. But it has had serious effects in large sections of the population. The body's natural nutrient-requirement signal, the appetite, has not evolved to cope with such unnatural foods. It knows when to stop us eating meat, but not when to stop us eating chocolate bars and cakes. It is also much easier to eat modern white bread than the stodgy, pre-industrial revolution bread.

During the past century there have been dramatic rises in a number of previously rare diseases. These include heart disease, cancers, diabetes, peptic ulcer, tooth decay, constipation and obesity. Although dietary fat is blamed for many of them, a half-century of research has failed consistently to provide any convincing evidence in support of this hypothesis. The fat-and-heart disease hypothesis relies on comparisons between disease patterns in 'civilised' countries and more primitive societies, and the amounts of fat in their respective diets. They purport to show that where a lot of fat is eaten there is a high incidence of heart disease, while others who eat less fat have lower incidences of the disease. However, if one makes similar comparisons, replacing fat with refined carbohydrate, one finds similar patterns. And in the case of refined carbohydrates, the case is much more compelling.

In 1935, Given pointed out a correlation between diabetes and carbohydrate intake. This has since been confirmed beyond doubt. A highly concentrated carbohydrate diet puts an immense strain on the pancreas to produce insulin. That is not to say that a largely plant-based diet will necessarily lead to diabetes. Many societies do have diets in which there is a large percentage of carbohydrate, yet do not suffer from diabetes. China and Ireland, where the principal food items were rice and potatoes respectively, had practically no diabetes. These diets, however, contained 'natural' unrefined carbohydrates. In Britain and the United States incidences of diabetes over the past century and during two great wars have followed very precisely the patterns of *refined* carbohydrate intake.

As far as obesity is concerned, it is very noticeable that in their natural environment, animals may vary in size, but never in shape: animals do not get fat. No rabbit gets fat by eating too much grass; no lion gets fat by eating too much antelope; no hawk gets fat by eating too many mice; no herring gets fat by eating too much plankton, and no wolf or wild dog gets fat from eating too many rabbits. Indeed, if we look around the natural animal kingdom, we find a striking absence of obesity in all species. It is also noticeably absent in primitive races of mankind. In 'civilised' man and his domesticated animals, however, obesity is all too common.

Dogs and cats

As a direct descendant of the wolf, the modern domestic dog is a pure carnivore. In its natural environment, it would catch and eat rabbits and other small mammals. Even if it were starving, it would never dream of eating wheat or digging up carrots. Man, however, has largely turned the dog into a herbivore. Meat is relatively expensive so the dog now survives largely on wheat, in the form of dog biscuits and bread. It is little wonder, therefore, that the domesticated dog suffers diseases that are totally unknown in its wild relatives. The domestic dog suffers exactly the same ills as civilised man: dental cavities, cancers, heart disease, hypertension, diabetes and, most noticeably, obesity.

The cat too is a pure carnivore and it too lives with man. However, the cat does not suffer the diseases of civilisation as the dog does. This is because the cat is an animal which 'does its own thing'. Although the cat enjoys the warmth of an open fire and a rug in front of it, it still hunts and eats mice and birds – its natural diet. Most prepared cat foods, unlike those for the dog, are also wholly meat- and fish-based. Thus, unlike the dog, a cat's life and diet are relatively natural. Indeed, the only time a domestic cat gets fat, or suffers other diseases, is when it is fed cat biscuits or other farinaceous food.

The diseases of Man

We can make similar comparisons between human cultures. McClellan and Du Bois pointed out that the Eskimos in Baffin Island and Greenland lived on a diet composed almost entirely of meat and fish, ate hardly any carbohydrate and suffered few diseases. This was not the case with the Labrador Eskimos. They had been 'civilised' and lived on preserved foods, dried potatoes, flour, canned foods and cereals. As a consequence, among them the diseases of civilisation were rife.

A comparison between the Masai tribes of East Africa, who live alongside the Kikuyu, shows a similar pattern. The Masai, when wholly carnivorous, were tall, healthy, long-lived and slim. The Kikuyu, when wholly vegetarian, were stunted, diseased, short-lived and pot-bellied. Over the last few decades, the Kikuyu have started to eat a mixed diet – and their health has improved. Since 1960 the Masai diet has also changed, but in the opposite direction. They are now eating less blood and meat, replacing it with maize and beans. Their health has deteriorated. The same is true of every primitive tribe which has had contact with 'civilisation'.

Overweight problems

Fats, proteins and carbohydrates can all be converted to glucose, a form of sugar which is used by the body as a source of energy. Fats contain approximately 9 calories per gram and proteins and carbohydrates have approximately 4 calories per gram each. The proteins and fats are essential in that they are used for purposes other than mere providers of energy. They are used to maintain and repair the body's cells, for example. Carbohydrates in the diet, however, have only one purpose – to be converted into glucose.

All slimmers know that sugar, above all else, is fattening. Every diet yet devised counsels quite rightly against eating sugar. But, in fact, the carbohydrates you eat, whether they are white crystals of sugar or starches found in cereals and vegetables when they enter your mouth, *all* turn to sugar in the body. Refined sugars and starches are used widely in pre-packed convenience foods. On packaged foods, the sugar content is frequently obscured by the manufacturers – sugar contents being variously described as: sucrose, fructose, glucose, maltose or dextrose. Bread, pasta, rice, and other cereals too, are all high in concentrated starches. So there is little point in keeping your consumption of sugar, the white granular stuff, low if you tuck in to packaged foods, bread and pasta.

The importance of blood-sugar levels

The main cause of overweight problems in the west is too high an intake of sugar and other sweet or starchy foods. When the body needs energy and blood sugar levels are low, the body signals to us the need to eat with the feeling of hunger. Then, if we are sensible, we eat a meal which is composed of food items which are digested and absorbed at different rates. This way energy is available continuously over the period to the next meal. When eaten, carbohydrates are digested and absorbed quickly, the proteins are digested more slowly and then the fats. If we eat the three in the correct proportions, there should be no problem. If the meal is too high in carbohydrates, however, the blood sugar level can rise quite rapidly. The body cannot use it as energy quickly enough and it is converted to fat and stored away. We put on weight. At the same time, the pancreas is secreting large amounts of insulin to reduce those high blood sugar levels, overcompensates, causing blood sugar to fall to a *low* level which makes us feel hungry again. So we eat more – and we tend then to snack on sweets! It is a vicious circle. We get hungry even though we eat more, get fat, run down and depressed.

The answer is to eat less of the carbohydrates so that the blood sugar level does not fluctuate so violently, coupled with an *increased* intake of fat. By taking longer to digest, fat not only prevents those violent fluctuations in blood-sugar levels, it gives a feeling of satiety, thus staving off the feelings of hunger for a longer time.

As you will have realised, it is not just slimmers who should beware of dietary carbohydrates. Apart from making us overweight, a number of other disorders are caused or exacerbated by too high an intake of sugars and starches – environmental diseases from diabetes and heart disease to decayed teeth and fatigue, and even virus diseases such as the common cold.

Sugar and heart disease

Despite the enormous amount of propaganda disseminated these days, we know that dietary animal fats and cholesterol are *not* responsible for the high incidence of heart disease in Western countries (see Chapter 6). There is a considerable body of evidence, however, that if there is a dietary cause, it is the carbohydrates we eat.

The heart muscle, like any other muscle in the body, needs certain nutrients in order to work correctly. The two chief energy-producing nutrients are oxygen and the blood-sugar, glucose, both of which are transported by the blood. These two react chemically to produce energy. As muscles work, lactic acid is produced as a waste product. This is normally carried away by the blood. Under certain circumstances, the lactic acid may accumulate abnormally in a muscle. If this happens in the heart muscle, it is responsible for heart pain. One condition which can cause such an abnormal accumulation is an abnormally low sugar utilisation by the heart muscle.

The cholesterol theory has it that blocked arteries prevent oxygen from reaching the heart muscle, but the majority of people who die of heart disease *do not have blocked coronary arteries*. The blocked artery hypothesis cannot account for this. However, the oxygen used in muscles to oxidise sugar is only half the equation. The low utilisation of sugar by the heart muscle may not be due to lack of oxygen but to low blood-sugar levels. And, as we saw above, low blood-sugar levels can be caused by a high-carbohydrate diet.

In the case of heart disease, both low blood-sugar and rapid fluctuations in blood-sugar levels are equally harmful. Eating a meal which has a high carbohydrate content first raises the blood-sugar levels quickly, then lowers it.

Triglycerides are fats found at high levels in many heart disease cases. Dietary fat is usually blamed, but blood triglyceride levels are proportional to sugar intake. Platelets, the agents which make blood clot when we are cut, also tend to clump together on a diet high in sugar. It has been shown that a diet which contains a large proportion of carbohydrate can cause blood clots and reduce the flow of blood to the extremities. If such a clot reaches the heart, it can be the cause of a coronary thrombosis. Reducing carbohydrate intake reduces the risk of a blood clot and, thus, of a heart attack.

Sugar and diabetes

Diabetes, or diabetes mellitus to give it its full title, is a disorder of carbohydrate metabolism in which sugars in the body are not oxidised to produce energy because the pancreas is unable to manufacture sufficient insulin. In this condition, blood-sugar levels become unstable. Diabetes damages the pancreas, kidneys and the retinas in the eyes, and increases susceptibility to heart disease. Avoiding sugar and refined carbohydrates, particularly in childhood, is the best way to avoid diabetes.

Thirty years ago, the diabetic would have been treated with a diet where 'The carbohydrate is reduced to a minimum and the fat increased to a maximum, consistent with no untoward symptoms'. Insulin was used only if diet failed. Strangely, today, it tends to be the other way round. The evidence against carbohydrates suggests that the old way was better.

Sugar and colds

Colds are looked upon as a fact of life – everyone gets them and they are not regarded as being serious. This concept may be incorrect. In 1954, the *British Medical Journal* published an article on respiratory infections as the cause of heart failure. It showed that respiratory infections, particularly colds, were the most common irritating and aggravating factors in congestive heart failure. In two studies of incidences of heart failure, more than half the patients had some form of respiratory infection and a direct relation was found between the frequent occurrence of heart failure and 'even minor colds'. Make no mistake, colds can be deadly.

Colds are caused by a virus. We probably all carry it, but we really do not need to 'catch a cold'. Colds occur only when the body's resistance is too weak to deal with them. Resistance is built up slowly over a long period of time but can be undermined easily. The common concept of catching a cold by going out in the rain, or getting cold is wrong. Getting tired and run down is much more likely to precipitate a cold. And so, it seems, is a diet that is high in sugars and cereal starches.

A study comparing the Kikuyu and Masai tribes demonstrated dramatically the role of carbohydrates in respiratory problems. The Kikuyu, who lived mainly on cereals, had a mortality from bronchitis and pneumonia which was 10 times as high as that of the meat-eating Masai. Another study at a girls' boarding school, found that the incidence of colds among the girls was directly related to the amount of sugar each consumed. The contention was that a high intake of sweets and other carbohydrates disposed the eater to a higher risk of respiratory problems such as colds. The advice given to reduce the likelihood of getting a cold was: cut out sugar and eat no bread or other products which contain either wheat or rye.

Sugar and mental illness and crime in children

Joseph Wilder, a New York doctor found, as long ago as 1943, that low blood-sugar levels in adults produced mental symptoms such as: depression, anxiety, irritability, slow mental processes, dullness and difficulty in making decisions. The effects of low blood-sugar in children were considerably more serious.

Children with this condition would be neurotic, psychopathic and have criminal tendencies, suffer anxiety, run away, be aggressive and destructive. Dr Wilder says: 'In its simplest form, it is the tendency to deny everything, contradict everything, refuse everything at any price . . . It is no wonder that a considerable number of criminal and semi-criminal acts have been observed in children in hypoglycaemic (low blood-sugar) states, ranging from destructiveness or violation of traffic regulations all the way to bestiality, arson and homicide.' The low blood-sugar/criminality link has been confirmed many times since.

Today, children are eating more sugar and sweetened foods than ever before in history – and, judging from reports in the press, committing more crimes. Could it be that the two are connected? Wilder realised that low blood-sugar was not caused by low intake of sugar, indeed that the reverse was the case. He said: 'Apparently, too copious feeding of sugar may, in the long run, cause an over-function of the islet cells of the pancreas and increase the tendency to hypoglycaemia; on the other hand, there are cases in which a diet extremely poor in carbohydrates and sugars may improve or even cure the condition.'

Sugar and tooth decay

Dental cavities are a fact of life today for many children. To strengthen children's teeth, we are all subjected to fluoridation of our water supplies. Yet fluoride is a very dangerous chemical. Dental cavities are not an inevitable consequence of childhood. As we saw earlier, they are caused by the food we eat; more precisely from the carbohydrates we eat. There is no doubt that sucrose, the white, refined table sugar, is by far the worst culprit. But it is not alone. Other sugars such as those found in processed foods are as bad, as are white bread and other cooked cereal products. Carbohydrate foods that are sticky enhance the effects even if eaten only infrequently. It is much healthier and safer to avoid the sweets than to risk fluoridation.

Sugar and hypertension

Salt intake is usually blamed for hypertension (high blood pressure), but this is another hypothesis that is not supported by the evidence. Clinical work at

Louisiana State University Medical School showed that sugar plays a part. Healthy kidneys are needed if hypertension is to be prevented. A high sugar load can damage the kidneys so that they cannot cope. This can lead to glucose intolerance, a condition which precedes such disorders as diabetes. Hypertension therefore, may be caused by dietary sugar, resulting in an inability by the body to process that sugar.

Conclusion

What we are advised to eat today is far removed from what we have adapted, and are genetically programmed to eat. Dieticians tell us to eat more bread, pasta, fruit and vegetables. All these are high in carbohydrates, and many in refined carbohydrates. For the most part, they are the carbohydrates in the diet which caused the damage listed above. Things like sugar, sticky sweets, soft drinks, pasta, cakes and white bread were the main culprits. But others which are harmful include dried fruits such as raisins and the starchier root vegetables. Cooked, refined, carbohydrate foods were worse than raw (but without cooking we could not eat them); green vegetables, which are generally low in carbohydrates, cooked or uncooked, present few problems.

Many of the disorders with which we are afflicted today, and which have a dietary cause, may fairly be laid at the door of our intake of refined and concentrated carbohydrates. There is no evidence that proteins are fattening or in any other way harmful, and no convincing evidence that fats from animal sources are either. We may need some carbohydrate in our diet but certainly not in large quantities, and not in the form that most is ingested. The best place to get the carbohydrate part of your diet is the greengrocer's shop – not the confectioner's, the baker's, or the grocer's shops.

The second rule is:
Reduce your intake of concentrated and refined carbohydrates.

3
SLIMMING CAN BE FATTENING

Slimming has been a factor in the lives of many people for generations. Over those years, slimming claims have been made for many specific items of food. Classic examples are grapefruit; pineapple or fibre. We have had inert fillers, low-calorie this, low-fat that. Then came a number of Low-Calorie Diets (LCDs) and Very Low Calorie Diets (VLCDs). There were even diets for diet haters. People lost weight – and put it on again. Many were harmed, some died.

As some women have realised that low-calorie dieting does not work, they have turned to more drastic measures. They have had their stomachs stapled so that they cannot eat so much, or had their jaws wired together so that all they can ingest is liquids, or had their small intestine shortened to reduce the amounts of energy it will absorb, or fat cells removed with liposuction. These are dangerous and drastic steps which, generally do not work. For example, one woman who had had her jaws wired, explained in an interview how she liquidised chocolate bars so that she could eat them. All these measures seem to achieve in the long run is a lot of pain and suffering followed by a loss of morale and self-esteem when they fail.

Eat less – weigh more
The extensive research carried out over many decades to answer the question of why some people, eating little, get fat and others remain thin no matter how much they eat, has concentrated on the simplistic idea that people get fat because they eat too much. What happens to food and how the body regulates its energy expenditure has been largely ignored. This has led in the main to the research being concentrated on trying to answer the wrong questions and it is no real surprise that it cannot find the right answers. In the meantime, the fatter

person is made out to be a glutton and is ridiculed by society.

But, hard though it may be to believe, people who are fat really do tend to eat *less* than those who are slim. That those who eat less are fatter than those who eat more was first suggested as long ago as 1961 and confirmed in several other studies since. In 1991, the latest study compared women who were 'small eaters' and others who were 'large eaters'. It found that although subjects classed as 'small eaters' ate, on average, less than 1,500 calories per day, they had an average 33% body fat, whereas the 'large eaters' eating around 2,400 calories per day, weighed significantly less and averaged only 22% body fat. Low-calorie slimming diets could actually be the cause of weight gain. Why should this be?

In the last chapter we looked at one reason that we become overweight – by eating the wrong food. This may, however, be coupled with another reason: overweight may also be caused by a malfunction of one or more of the body's energy-regulating organs brought about, in most cases, by a protracted period of eating less than the body needs.

Energy regulation systems

There is little doubt that most cases of corpulence are caused initially by the sorts of food that we eat. The reason we, as a nation, are getting fatter is because of the advice we have been getting from food companies, slimming magazines and dieticians. Only eat as many calories as your body uses, we are told. How can we do this? We cannot possibly measure by mental arithmetic our energy input to the nearest calorie and tailor our workload to use up exactly the same amount as we put in.

However, the body has mechanisms which can. The systems which regulate food input and energy output are complex but are completely self-regulatory. They rely on numerous interacting neuro-chemical or opiate systems (which were discovered as recently as 1975) and brown fat.

To understand how to obtain and retain a correct weight successfully, it may be helpful to understand something of the body's natural regulatory controls. We must understand how different types of food are dealt with by the body, and how the body regulates energy input/output. The amount we eat and what we eat may have a profound effect on the systems which regulate why and when we eat, as well as what happens to food after we have eaten it. You are an individual and are different from other individuals. You have a different body, lead a different life, have a different job and different hobbies, hopes and worries. Your energy needs are not necessarily the same as those of your peers.

How can you know how much of any nutrient your body needs? The answer is, you cannot. But, your body can and, if you are aware of it, your body can tell you.

The control systems may be divided into two: those which regulate energy input and those which regulate energy output, the two working together to achieve a balance.

On the energy input side, the controls are hunger and appetite. As your blood-sugar levels fall, and energy is required, you begin to feel hungry. This feeling of hunger is your body's way of telling you to eat. In tandem with hunger comes appetite. As the various bodily processes take place, different nutrients are used and energy is expended. All must be replaced in the correct proportions. It is with appetite that the body tells you what combination of proteins, fats, and carbohydrates to eat. Without hunger you would not know when to eat and without appetite you would not know what to eat. These are the signals with which your body communicates with you. They measure and time the body's needs very precisely. If these signals are not heeded, body needs are not met and permanent damage can result.

All three food groups can be converted for use as energy but they convert at different rates. Carbohydrates are broken down quickest followed by the proteins and, lastly, the fats. The correct combination is required to supply energy at a constant rate.

As food is eaten, it is assessed by sensors in the upper gut. These set up a chain of electro-chemical reactions involving the gut opiates. These opiates are similar to morphine in their properties but much stronger. Most are in the intestinal nerve cells, others in the part of the brain which regulates appetite. These opiates control feelings of hunger and the appetite. As food is eaten other sensors in the upper gut assess its nutritional suitability as a meal and the body's requirement for particular nutrients. As they are supplied, the appetite for them diminishes until, eventually, the appetite is satisfied and it 'switches off' the appetite for that nutrient. When all needs are met, we no longer feel hungry and we stop eating.

The body's use of energy, the output side of the body's energy balance, is controlled by our brown fat. Although mainly located in the upper back, there are clusters of brown fat cells in many parts of the body. Their job is to regulate the amount of energy the body uses. Brown fat is a special fat that is fundamentally different from ordinary white fat both in composition and function. White fat is mainly an energy storage system where excess calories are deposited. Brown fat, on the other hand, is an energy-using material which is stimulated by the nervous system to burn up calories. Thus brown fat reduces the amount of white fat. Brown fat's primary task is to regulate and maintain our body temperature. As it uses energy much faster than other body cells, it is used to produce warmth in cold weather. When this warmth is not required it is dissipated. Brown fat also plays an important role in weight control by burning off excess calories.

The rhythm method of girth control

Most slimming diets today say that to lose weight one must eat fewer calories (energy) than one uses. The theory explains that if one puts in more fuel than is burnt, the excess must go somewhere and we get fat. If we were cars, that might be so but we are not cars. Using the control outlined above, the healthy body can regulate very precisely the rate at which it uses fuel in conjunction with the amount ingested. When we eat less than our appetite says we need, the first effect is that the appetite is not satisfied. This is abnormal and unnatural. If we continue, the appetite becomes blunted until eventually it no longer works correctly.

At the same time, if our energy intake is insufficient, we start to use up our energy stores and lose weight. But if our energy intake continues to be less than we need, the brown fat recognises that we are starving and reduces its activity. It conserves energy by slowing down the rate at which the body uses it. This is why at the start of a diet, weight loss may be high but then, as we continue with it, weight loss gets progressively less. When we resume a 'normal' eating pattern, after the period of dieting, the body takes the opportunity to store a little extra in case of more lean times to come, and a little more weight is put on. This is why most people who diet get progressively fatter over the years. This process leads to ever more stringent diets, the brown fat is damaged, it atrophies and stops working. The more you diet, the worse it gets, and the fatter you will get.

The pattern, then, is that the dieter changes from one diet to another, and periods of dieting are alternated with periods of normal eating. This produces a 'yo-yo' effect which weakens the weight-regulating mechanisms, making it necessary for the dieter to undertake ever more stringent diets to achieve the same weight loss.

Persistent low-calorie dieting can damage any of the control systems. Many people crave food all day. In them there is damage to the switch-off opiates, their appetite has become defective and they are never satisfied. These are the people who cannot help nibbling between meals. There are others who get fat and yet they eat very little – and they have great difficulty in convincing their doctors of this. Here it is the activation of their brown fat which is at fault.

Eventually, both the opiate and the brown fat systems may become flawed. If one persists with such diets and the brown fat is deactivated for any length of time, it can atrophy and become progressively less able to fulfil its regulatory function. When the brown fat is defective, people get and remain overweight no matter how little they eat. This is why it is dangerous to try to slim unnecessarily; the body's energy-regulating systems are damaged and fashion-conscious women who did not really need to lose weight in the first place, end up with an intractable weight problem. The longer it goes on the worse it gets and obesity is the inevitable result.

Low-calorie dietary regimes not only invariably fail, they also damage the health, engender a feeling of disillusion and failure, lower the morale and increase mental as well as physical stress. They are damaging both physically and mentally.

Normalisation of controls

For the natural controls to work correctly they must be normalised. Appetite and hunger are natural and vital signals and both must be satisfied. Modern low-calorie diets are abnormal. They encourage hunger but do not satisfy it. Neither, usually, do they satisfy the appetite. Thus these mechanisms are harmed. The most important prerequisite of any diet, therefore, is to get the body's systems working normally again. If you are comparatively new to dieting, this should not be too big a problem. It may take a little longer if you have been low-calorie dieting for many years. Nevertheless, it is never too late to begin eating properly.

The third rule, therefore, is:
**If you are overweight, use a slimming
diet that does not restrict calories.**

And the fourth rule is:
Never try to lose more than 2 pounds in weight per week.

A lie is halfway round the world before truth has got its boots on. Mark Twain

4
EXERCISE AS A SLIMMING AID

'Fitness' is a billion-pound industry which promotes books, exercise machinery, weights, clothing and expensive venues. Exercise psychologists make nice livings for themselves by tailoring 'body building', 'body awareness' and 'personalised' programmes for the individual. The industry uses every trick of the advertising trade to promote this lucrative business. Emotive issues such as obesity, heart disease and the implication that to be unfit is to be inferior, are used to good effect in promoting all sorts of dubious gadgets and products.

But fitness is not a scientific term and has no scientific method of measurement. All healthy people are fit people. When told that one needs to exercise, one should take into consideration the commercial bias of the person giving the advice.

Exercise and slimming

Sport and exercise of the right kind can be rewarding both as a social outlet and in terms of feeling good. As such they have an important role to play, particularly as leisure-time for most of us is increasing. However, as a means of losing weight, exercise is useless.

Certainly, it is possible to lose some weight by exercising. But weight so lost is costly, transient, potentially dangerous and self-defeating. Firstly, if the amount of energy expended in exercise is less than the amount readily available for use in the body, no body fat will be used. Secondly, if more energy is expended than is available, that energy supply is exhausted and any weight loss is at a cost of stress on the body. In an attempt to conserve energy, the body tries to slow down. The formula is another form of calorie manipulation similar to eating less energy (calories) than one uses. Increasing energy-output with exercise is the same as decreasing energy-input with a low-calorie diet – and the overall effect will be the same.

One is again eating less than one needs and, no matter how long the exercise is continued, as soon as one stops, weight is put on again. The effect is most noticeable when the non-athlete performs bouts of exhaustive exercise every two or three days. Any lost weight will be replaced between one bout and the next.

In a way similar to dieting, the effect on the body's brown fat is that its action is temporarily switched off and if this inaction is continued for any length of time, it becomes less and less able to fulfil its function. The effects are as dangerous as dieting in the long term.

Lastly, exercise exhaustive enough to cause a weight loss has other serious side effects, particularly on women. If such exercise is undertaken before or around the age of puberty, the menarche may be delayed by as much as 2 or 3 years. In fact, each year of intensive athletic training before the menarche can delay it by an average of 5 months. Later, it is also the cause of amenorrhoea (cessation of periods) which can persist even after weight is regained, abnormal menstrual cycles, abnormal sex hormone patterns and impaired reproductive function. These are the effects on as many as 50% of women indulging in such activities, and so should be an important consideration in those wishing to have a family. But is not just women who are affected by such exercise regimes. In men too there are similar effects, with reduced testosterone (the male sex hormone) found in long-distance runners.

The dubious hypothesis that exhaustive exercise produces fitness has led to a new medical term referred to in the *Lancet* as 'the morbid exercise syndrome'. It describes a condition whereby what started usually as a last desperate attempt to lose weight turns into an obsession where the participant cannot stop exercising even when he or she becomes injured – a sort of anorexia nervosa.

The dangers of too much exercise

For anyone contemplating taking up the more strenuous forms, the advice from the *American Heart Journal* is:

'Be tested and have an exercise programme devised after clinical trials and tests on the heart as, although regular exercise will lower the overall risk of cardiovascular disease, there is a statistically significant increase in the risk of sudden death'.

There are real risks if those who are not seasoned athletes attempt to emulate them, to break through the pain barrier, or as Jane Fonda puts it, 'go for the burn'. While seasoned athletes with their increased oxygenating capacity may be able to prolong their muscular activity before the onset of pain, the average mortal cannot and, indeed, should not attempt to emulate them. The risk to health and even life is unacceptably high. Over the past few years there have been reports of significant numbers of cases of sudden death in healthy young men out jogging or playing squash because they disregarded the pain barrier.

There has also been a vast number of cases of broken bones, dislocations, and damage to internal organs, muscles, tendons and ligaments. A study from Japan cited a 25% incidence of injury in those undertaking exhaustive exercise and these figures are confirmed in similar Western studies. The pain barrier is the body's way of saying that its limit of toleration has been reached. Disregarding this message is foolhardy.

Exercise-induced allergies are also on the increase. These include asthma, skin itching and urticaria (nettle rash). Also increasing are cases of cardiovascular collapse and respiratory obstruction. While some conditions may be relatively minor annoyances, others are definitely life-threatening, typically affecting teenagers and young adults. The usual trigger for an attack is running, but some patients have collapsed after only a brisk walk. It is not possible to predict an attack even among people with a history of such attacks whilst running, and even joggers who have been running for many years without incident frequently collapse. Unfortunately, most of those affected, even those with the life-threatening attacks, seem reluctant to discontinue their exercise programmes. They are lucky that in most cases treatment is possible and the treatments are improving. Nevertheless, current advice to joggers is: never jog alone.

Incidentally, athletes are not known for their longevity.

In spite of the risks, or more probably because people are not made aware of them, many adopt exercise programmes which involve sudden intensive exertion such as squash or 'aerobics'.

The term 'aerobics' means using oxygen and it is claimed that aerobic exercise is beneficial because it increases the amount of oxygen in the body tissues. In fact, the strenuous exercise demanded can increase the oxygen demand to a point where that demand cannot be met and, far from increasing tissue oxygenation, it decreases it. There are two points to be made here. Firstly, the type of exercise outlined above brings into play the body's emergency system. In case of an emergency, of course, it would be justified.

However, this self-inflicted trauma brought upon the body without cause is an unnecessary risk to health. Also, the body has regulatory systems which control very accurately the amount of oxygen it needs. A programme to get extra oxygen into the body is not only superfluous, it is dangerous. Excess oxygen is as dangerous as a deficit. That was demonstrated tragically some years ago when many babies were blinded by its over-enthusiastic use.

The body's emergency system, whether it is activated by the need to run away from danger or to stay and fight, or as a result of strenuous exercise, causes a number of automatic responses which prepare the body to face the danger to come. Amongst these, the heart beat is accelerated and minor blood vessels are constricted so that more blood is fed to the brain and muscles and the lungs take in more oxygen. Blood levels of cholesterol are increased. Adrenalin is pumped into the bloodstream helping these changes, stopping or slowing the digestive process, and stimulating the conversion of glycogen, a form of sugar stored by the body, into glucose which the body can use more easily as a source of energy.

In an emergency, the individual can escape from the threat or destroy it and the body can return to normal. In the case of prolonged physical exertion, however, the body is forced to continue, setting in motion a series of changes called the General Adaption Syndrome. A major and important change is the prolonged production of a group of adrenal hormones called corticosteroids. An excessive production of corticosteroids has been shown to produce heart disease, hypertension and stomach ulcers. It can damage the immune system harming the body's ability to fight infectious diseases and cancer. Depletion of the corticosteroids may also cause rheumatoid arthritis.

Conclusion

Exercise has its part to play in a normal healthy lifestyle. However, it is possible to overdo it – particularly if you are not used to it – and this can be dangerous. By all means use exercise as a social activity or as means of toning muscles. It is even possible to slim slightly, but it is of no use at all as a weight-reducing aid.

There was an old man of Tobago,
Who lived on rice, gruel and sago;
'Til much to his bliss,
His physician said this –
To a leg, sir, of mutton you may go.
R S Sharpe, circa 1822

5
THE HISTORY OF SLIMMING

Food can be divided into three groups: carbohydrates, proteins and fats. All of them provide energy (calories): fats have approximately 9 calories per gram and proteins and carbohydrates roughly 4 calories per gram each. Any of them, therefore, will provide the body with the energy it needs. But the body needs nutrients other than energy and this is where the three types of food differ.

Carbohydrates provide only energy. They have none of the essential components that the body needs to build or repair its tissues. A person fed only carbohydrates would starve to death no matter how much he ate. His body would break down other body proteins, such as muscle, in an attempt to keep the essential organs functioning. At the same time he would put on weight while he died as the carbohydrate surplus was stored as body fat. Carbohydrates are found in abundance in foods of vegetable origin.

Proteins are essential to the body, providing the material from which body cells are made and repaired. These are required on a daily basis. Although the calorie density of proteins is the same as that of carbohydrates, you will have noticed that slimming diets do not restrict the intake of proteins. This is because it has been realised since the 1930s that protein has a slimming effect. Proteins are composed of amino acids, of which there are twenty-three. Eight of these are essential, the body can manufacture the rest.

Complete proteins, that is those which contain all the essential amino acids in the correct proportions, are found in meats, fish, eggs and dairy products and also soyabean used as tempeh or tofu.

Incomplete proteins have some but not all essential amino acids. Sources of incomplete proteins are: cereals, nuts, seeds and legumes.

By far the best sources of protein are animal products. Although it is

44

possible to combine the various sources of incomplete proteins to supply all the essential amino acids on a vegetarian diet, this would lead inevitably to a high intake of carbohydrates.

Fat has more than twice as much energy as carbohydrate. Yet we are taught to regard carbohydrate as the primary source of energy. But fat is more than just the best energy source. It also contains: lipids which are used in the brain and nervous system, without which we become irritable and aggressive; sterols, precursors of a number of hormones (including the sex hormones); and the fat-soluble vitamins A, D, E and K. These vitamins can be found in other foods, but without the presence of dietary fat, the body cannot absorb them. People who are forced to eat lean meat such as rabbit and who are unable to obtain fat from other sources, develop diarrhoea and headache within only a few days. If they continue for any length of time, they become incapable of working.

The body also requires vitamins, minerals and trace elements. The western diet provides all these in abundance so long as a mixed diet is eaten. We will not concern ourselves with them as there is no risk of deficiency except on vegetarian diets or those which are high in bran fibre. Neither type will be advocated here.

The Banting Diet

Since the dawn of recorded history, the most prized food was fat. Until the second half of the twentieth century, fat was not believed to be unhealthy; quite the opposite. But with imperfect knowledge, it was thought to be the cause of the excessive weight gain in Western countries and so, for the overweight only, fat was to be avoided.

In 1862, however, a layman was to start a process which should have changed western medical thinking on diet radically. In that year, 66-year-old William Banting (the Duke of Wellington's coffin maker) weighed 202 pounds and he was only 5ft.5in tall. He was too fat to tie his own shoelaces and had to come downstairs backwards to avoid jarring his knees.

The first slimming advice had been given to him when he began to get fat in his thirties. This advice was to increase 'bodily exertion before any ordinary daily labours began'. He took up rowing in a heavy boat for two hours a day – and put on weight! He was advised to stop rowing.

After that he tried sea air and swimming, walking, and riding. He drank 'gallons of physic and liquor potassae', took the waters at Leamington, Cheltenham and Harrogate, and tried starvation diets. He was in hospital 20 times in as many years for weight reduction – all in vain. He took Turkish baths at a rate of three a week for the first fifty and then less frequently up to eighty but lost only 6 lbs in all that time, and had less and less energy. He gave up.

By August of 1862 Banting had started to go deaf so he visited an ear, nose and throat specialist, Dr. William Harvey FRCS. Harvey recognised that the cause of Banting's deafness was his obesity and put him on a diet. By Christmas, Banting was down to 184 lbs and by the following August 156 lbs. Not only had his hearing been restored, he had lost nearly 50 lbs in weight and 12¼ inches off his waist. Banting was delighted. He would have gone through hell to achieve this reduction but it had not been necessary.

We know what this miraculous diet was because in 1863, Banting published his *Letter on Corpulence* in which he tells us. It was a high-protein, high-fat, low-carbohydrate diet. Harvey's advice to him was to give up foods which 'contain starch and saccharine matter' – and it worked. His diet consisted of:

BREAKFAST. 4-5 ounces beef, mutton, kidneys, broiled fish, bacon or cold meat of any kind except pork (at that time pork was thought to contain carbohydrates); a large cup of tea (without milk or sugar), a little biscuit or one ounce of dry toast.

DINNER. 5-6 ounces of fish, or meat, any vegetables except potato, one ounce of dry toast, fruit of any pudding (not the pastry), any kind of poultry or game, and 2-3 glasses of good claret, sherry or Madeira. Champagne, port and beer were forbidden.

TEA. 2-3 ounces of fruit, a rusk or two and a cup of tea without milk or sugar.

SUPPER. 3-4 ounces of meat or fish, similar to dinner, with a glass or two of claret.

NIGHTCAP. Tumbler of grog – gin, whisky or brandy (without sugar) or a glass or two of claret or sherry.

By today's reckoning this would come to some 2,800 calories per day. And on this diet Banting lost approx 1lb per week from August 1862 to August 1863. In his own words he says: 'I can confidently state that quantity of diet may safely be left to the natural appetite; and that it is quality only which is essential to abate and cure corpulence.' He also said:

'I can conscientiously assert I never lived so well as under the new plan of dietary, which I should have formerly thought a dangerous, extravagant trespass upon health.'

'It is simply miraculous.'

'These important desiderata have been attained by the most easy and comfortable means, with but little medicine, and almost entirely by a system of diet, that formerly I should have thought dangerously generous.'

In a later edition of *Letter on Corpulence* he says: 'If bread is the staff of life, it is also the prime cause of obesity.'

When Banting's letter in which he described the diet and its amazing results was published, it so went against the established doctrine that it set up a howl of protest among members of the medical profession. The 'Banting Diet' became the centre of a bitter controversy and Banting's papers and book were ridiculed and distorted. No one could deny that the diet worked, but as it was published by a layman, and the medical men were anxious that their position in society should not be undermined, they felt bound to attack it. Banting's paper was criticized solely on the grounds that it was unscientific.

Harvey had a problem too. He had an effective treatment for obesity but not a convincing theory to explain it. As he was a medical man and so easier for the other members of his profession to attack, he came in for a great deal of ridicule until, in the end, his practice began to suffer.

However, the public were impressed. Many desperate, overweight people tried the diet, and found that it worked. Like it or not, the medical profession could not ignore it. This obvious success meant that the Banting Diet had to be explained somehow. To the rescue came a Dr. Felix von Niemeyer of Stuttgart who managed to make it acceptable with a total shift in its philosophy. At that time, the theory was that carbohydrates and fat burned together in the lungs to produce heat. The two were called respiratory foods. Von Niemeyer's answer to the doctors' problem was simple. Everyone knew that protein was not fattening -- only the respiratory foods, fats and carbohydrates. He, therefore, interpreted 'meat' to mean only lean meat and that solved the problem. The Banting Diet became a high protein diet with both carbohydrate and fat restricted and, with this modification, it became very popular; the phrase 'to bant' coming to mean to slim. Thus the overeating dogma became enshrined in history and still forms the basis of slimming diets today.

Banting's descriptions of the diet are quite clear, however. Nowhere is there any instruction to remove the fat from the meat, nowhere does he tell us to avoid butter and there was no restriction on the total quantity of food which could be taken. Only carbohydrate was restricted. He always maintained that Dr. von Niemeyer's altered diet was far inferior to the one that had so changed his life. Banting, incidentally, lived to the age of 81 in physical comfort and remained at a normal weight.

The Banting diet is confirmed

Banting's publication of his diet travelled widely. In the 1890s, an American doctor, Helen Densmore, modelled diets on Banting. She tells how she and her patients lost an average 10-15 lbs in the first month on the diet and then 6-8 lbs in subsequent months 'by a diet from which bread, cereals and starchy food were excluded'. Her advice to would-be slimmers was: 'One pound of beef or mutton or fish per day with a moderate amount of the non-starchy vegetables given above (tomatoes, lettuce, string beans, spinach and such) will be found ample for any obese person of sedentary habits.'

Dr Densmore was scathing of those others of her profession who derided Banting's diet. She says of them: 'Those very specialists who are at this time prospering greatly by the reduction of obesity and who are indebted to Mr Banting for all their prosperity are loud, nevertheless, in their condemnation of the Banting method.'

In 1906, Dr. Vilhjalmur Stefansson, who later became a world-famous explorer and anthropologist, revolutionized polar exploration by crossing the Arctic alone and living off the land with the Eskimos. It was not quite what had been planned. He had gone on ahead of the Leffingwell-Mikkelson Expedition and had missed a planned rendezvous. He was left to spend an Arctic winter with the Eskimos eating a diet composed only of meat and fish. Unlike the diet he had been brought up on, it contained no plant material whatsoever. On this regime, Stefansson remained in perfect health and did not get fat.

Some time after this experience, Dr. Stefansson returned to the Arctic with a colleague, Dr. Karsten Anderson, to carry out research for the American Museum of Natural History. They were supplied with every necessity including a year's supply of 'civilized' food but they elected instead to live off the land. In the end, the one-year project stretched to four, during which time the two men ate only the meat they could kill and the fish they could catch. They discovered that, during one period when they were forced to eat lean caribou meat and could get no seal oil, they became ill, but as soon as they managed to find fat, they recovered. Neither of the two men suffered any ill effects whatsoever from their four-year experiment.

It was evident to Stefansson, as it had been to Banting, that the body could function perfectly well, remain healthy, vigorous and slender if it used a diet in which as much food could be eaten as the body required, the total number of calories could be ignored and only carbohydrate was restricted.

In 1928, Stefansson and Anderson entered Bellevue Hospital, New York for a controlled experiment into the effects of an all-meat diet on the body. The committee which was assembled to supervise the experiment was one of the best qualified in medical history, consisting as it did of the leaders of all the branches of science related to the subject. The experiment was designed to find the answer to a number of questions about which there was some debate:

1. Does the withholding of vegetable foods cause scurvy?
2. Will an all-meat diet cause other deficiency diseases?
3. Will it cause mineral deficiencies, of calcium in particular?
4. Will it have a harmful effect on the heart, blood vessels or kidneys?
5. Will it promote the growth of harmful bacteria in the gut?

The results of the year-long trial were published in 1930 in the *Journal of Biological Chemistry* and showed that the answer to all of the questions was 'no'. There were no deficiency problems; they remained perfectly healthy; their bowels remained normal, except that their stools were smaller and did not smell. The absence of carbohydrate from their diet appeared to have only good effects.

One interesting finding from a heart disease point of view was that Stefansson's blood cholesterol level *fell* by 51 mg (1.3 mmol/l) while he was on the all-meat diet, rising again at the end of the study when he returned to a mixed diet. His intake had varied between 2,000 and 3,100 calories per day and he derived, by choice, an average of 80% of his energy from animal fat and the other 20% from protein.

But the published results had little effect. A diet which allowed as much meat as one could eat and also allowed a large proportion of fat must contain lots of calories. To the public, lots of calories meant putting on weight.

In 1944, another famous experiment was carried out by Dr. B F Donaldson at the New York Hospital when very overweight patients were reduced on high-fat, low-carbohydrate diets. The patients were encouraged to eat as much as they wanted and some of the sceptical ones certainly did – and they lost weight. High-fat, high-protein, low-carbohydrate diets were back. In Britain, deeply involved in a war and with food rationed, however, this experiment went largely unnoticed. Even in America, the average slimmer went on counting the calories in her low-calorie salad oblivious of the harm she was doing to her health.

Just after the Second World War, the E I du Pont chemical company of America undertook a slimming programme with some of its overweight executives who had had no success with the more usual low-calorie diets. The programme was run by Dr. A W Pennington and the director of du Pont's medical division, Dr. G H Gehrmann. Pennington had sifted through all the available evidence and decided on Banting's recommendations. Therefore, the subjects were allowed all the protein and fat they wanted, with carbohydrates withheld, and the results were spectacular. Averaged out, each of the dieters lost 22 lbs in three months. And calorie intake averaged 3,000 per day!

This time the public were interested and *Holiday* magazine published a series about the project. But the regimen offered so many calories and the general public had been so brainwashed for so long, that most found it impossible to believe that such a diet could work.

In 1956 Professor A Kekwick and Dr. G L S Pawan tested and evaluated Banting's diet scientifically at the Middlesex Hospital in London. They opined that if weight loss in overweight persons was merely a case of reducing dietary calorie intake to below the amount the body needed, then the lower the intake of calories, the greater should be the weight loss. To show this they used diets of 500, 1,000, 1,500 and 2,000 calories made up of constant proportions of carbohydrates (47%), proteins (20%) and fat (33%). This first series of tests, not surprisingly, did find a definite relation between the deficiency of calories and the amount of weight lost.

They went on to reason that if a deficiency in calorie intake alone was responsible for weight loss, then diets of equal calorific value, regardless of composition, should produce equal loss of weight. To test this, a second series of tests, where all the diets were 1,000 calories, should prove it. Thus three 1,000 calorie diets were formulated. These were 90% carbohydrate, or 90% protein or 90% fat respectively plus a fourth which was a normal mixed diet. So different were the rates of weight loss in this series of tests, that it was obvious that the *composition* of the diet was far more important than simply the intake of calories. Several of those on the 1,000-calorie carbohydrate diet actually gained weight. And subjects on the high-fat diet lost very much more than those on the others.

As it seemed that it was the composition of the diet that had the most profound effect on weight loss when the diets were restricted to below what the body needed, a third series of tests was performed. In these, patients were put on 2,000-calorie diets with a normal composition of protein, fat and carbohydrate. During this test, the patients either maintained their weight or gained slightly. Their calorie intakes were then increased to 2,600 and the composition of the diets was altered by increasing the amount of fat and protein and reducing the amount of carbohydrate. This time the patients lost weight.

There could be only one explanation: 'The composition of the diet can alter the expenditure of calories in obese persons – increasing it when proteins and fat are given and decreasing it when carbohydrates are given.'

Kekwick and Pawan's conclusions were summarised in the September 1957 edition of *Metabolism, Clinical and Experimental*. It said: 'If the proportions of fat, proteins and carbohydrate were kept constant, the rate of weight loss was then proportional to the calorie intake. If the calorie intake was kept constant, however, at 1,000 calories per day, the most rapid weight loss was noted with high fat diets . . . But when the calorie intake was raised to 2,600 daily in these patients, weight loss would still occur provided that this intake was given mainly in the form of fat and protein.'

These findings came as no surprise as far as dietary protein was concerned. The dynamic action of protein in weight loss had been known for many years. It did come as a surprise, however, that fat also worked in this way; particularly as the slimming action of dietary fat appeared to be greater than that of protein.

It should not have been a surprise, however, as similar findings had also been published the previous year by Hausberger and Milstein at Jefferson Medical College in the USA. In their experiments too, the greater the amount of fat in the diet, the greater was the weight loss. They had tested 4 diets which were: high in fat (Diet A), high in carbohydrate (Diet C), or in protein (Diet D), plus a 'normal' diet (Diet B). The compositions of the diets are tabled below:

Table I: *Composition of test diets in grams per 100 grams*

	Fat	Carb	Protein
Diet A.	60	1.2	26
Diet B.	35	34	15
Diet C	13	55	15
Diet D.	0.8	15	70

They found that subjects did not put on weight during prolonged fasting or while eating diet A (high-fat). 'This diet resembles the quantitative composition of the metabolic fuels which are used by the organism during fasting.' All the other diets, however, did cause some weight gain. Diet B, containing equal amounts of fat and carbohydrate, caused a small increase in body fat. Diet C, high in carbohydrates, caused a greater increase in body fat. Diet D, which was practically fat free, however, caused by far the greatest weight gain in subjects.

In a nutshell, the research which had been carried out showed that a high-fat diet stopped the formation of body fat and that the greatest increase in body fat formation was noticed on a high-carbohydrate, fat-free diet. Nevertheless, it is still this latter type of diet which is recommended to slimmers today!

All these experiments showed that eating fat actually speeded up weight loss. Doctors now had justification to base slimming diets on reduction of carbohydrate only rather than either a reduction of carbohydrates and fat or a restriction of total calories. The overweight need never feel hungry again. Fats need not, indeed should not, be reduced as they have an important satiety value as well as being a valuable source of essential nutrients.

But by the late 1950s, fat began to be suspected of being implicated in the rising incidence of coronary heart disease. Doctors began to think twice before advocating diets which were high in fat, balancing the risks associated with being excessively overweight with the risk of heart disease. Banting's low-carbohydrate, high-fat, diet began to go out of fashion. By the mid-1970s, to all intents it was dead.

Modern slimming diets

Banting's diet, which had no calorie restriction, had always been out of step with all other diets. It worked, and this meant that people using it did not become fat and did not need to spend money continually struggling to stay slim. When the fat diet/heart disease risk was hypothesised, however, all that changed. People could be exploited again. Thus, all modern diets have returned to the discredited early-19th-century theory, relying on one overriding philosophy: If you are overweight, you must be eating more calories than you are using. All modern diets, therefore, work on only one principle: cut down. In effect, you starve. And in that is the recipe for failure.

The demise of the Banting diet allowed an explosion of diets. In 1967, *The Doctor's Quick Weight Loss Diet* was published. This gave a diet on which the author claimed weight losses of up to 13 pounds per week. It allowed only lean meats and fish, cottage and skim milk cheeses, and water – no fat and no carbohydrates. In 1978 *The Complete Scarsdale Medical Diet*, co-authored by the same author as the previous book, gave a similar diet. This time it claimed to be able to cause the loss of 20 pounds in two weeks. We know that sustained weight loss of over about 2 pounds a week is a serious threat to health. Both these diets are seriously deficient in a number of vitamins and essential minerals.

The Pritikin diet appeared in 1979, firstly as *The Pritikin Program* and later as the *Maximum Weight Loss Diet*. This was written by Nathan Pritikin, an electronic engineer. This vegetarian-based, fat-free diet was not just a slimming diet but one which, it was claimed, would promote a long life. On it, a dieter was allowed to eat as many raw vegetables as he liked. It looked like an unlimited-calorie diet but, as raw vegetables are extremely low in calories, it too was in reality a low-calorie diet and doomed to failure. It was not much of a success as a life-prolonging diet either, at least to its originator – Pritikin committed suicide in February 1985. Undeterred by this setback, his son Robert, director of The Pritikin Longevity Center published T*he New Pritikin Program* in 1990. Such diets which are low in fat cause brain disturbances and severe emotional changes. They lead to depression, anxiety and frustration. They also reduce significantly the body's resistance to disease and can ultimately lead to chronic ill health.

Next in line was the infamous *Beverly Hills Diet* which was published in 1981. The author, who trained in drama, bases the diet on food-combining. That is, eating foods which do not 'fight one another, digestively speaking'. As she claims that proteins and carbohydrates 'fight', they should not be eaten together. It is a bizarre notion. Equally bizarre is her belief that enzymes which digest carbohydrates fight with those which digest proteins. This fighting, she says, causes food to remain undigested and get 'stuck' in the body. It is accumulations of food stuck in this way, she maintains, that make us put on weight. The claim is that if foods are combined properly so that they do not fight, they will be processed properly and we will not gain weight. It is, of course, utter nonsense. All undigested food passes through and out of the body. It is only fully digested food which can be absorbed and cause fatness. The Beverly Hills diet also advocates the eating of fruits such as papaya and pineapple as it claims that they have 'fat burning enzymes' which work on body fat. This again is arrant nonsense – fruit enzymes are proteins which are broken down in the gut long before they get anywhere near fatty tissue. Such a diet as this is much more likely to cause severe diarrhoea and mineral loss. In a later book, the author refers to the Beverly Hills Diet in terms of the Chinese Yin and Yang philosophy. This is the basis of the extreme Zen Macrobiotic Diet which is so nutritionally unbalanced as to cause scurvy, kidney failure and death.

The Beverly Hills Diet was a one-type-of-food-only diet. There were several others including the banana-only diet, the fish-only diet, the juices-only diet and the yogurt-only diet. The next diet that came along in 1982, the *F-Plan Diet*, was also based on one ingredient. In this case it was not a food but the non-food, dietary fibre. Audrey Eyton's F-Plan effectively doubles the intake of dietary fibre by adding bran to just about everything. This, she says, gives a feeling of fullness and a consequent loss of appetite. But this feeling is distinctly ephemeral. Bran moves through the gut faster than real food and the effect is soon lost. The mechanisms in the duodenum also recognise that what is passing has little nutritional content and the appetite is switched on again. It is not the fibre in the F-Plan Diet which does the work. The F-Plan is just like all the others – a low-calorie diet. Eyton admits this. She states in her book: 'Never let anyone, or any diet, convince you that calories don't count in achieving weight loss. They do. They are what slimming is all about.'

Cellulite – the truth

After puberty, women's thighs tend to develop an 'orange peel' effect. This is caused by fat. You do not have to be overweight for this to happen – it happens to slim women as well and it is perfectly natural. The phenomenon is restricted to women as part of the process of coming to sexual maturity. This store of fat, for that is what it is, prepares a woman for childbearing. But it can be unsightly and women do not like it. Fat in this part of the body was given the name 'cellulite' by a French cosmetic company as an advertising ploy in order to sell its products. And so began a myth.

Women are told that cellulite is a store of the body's waste material. Rosemary Conley in her book, *Complete Hip and Thigh Diet*, talking about constipation states: 'if the waste matter is not leaving the body through the normal channels the body will store it away from the bloodstream and again the islands of fat cells causing cellulite provide the perfect storehouse'. I find it hard to believe that, if a woman does not go to the lavatory, her body will deposit its waste in her legs! As a man, I wonder where mine would go?

The removal of cellulite has become the goal of many a slimmer. The problem is that women generally do not want to lose weight from their busts at the same time. This has led to dietary regimes which are so selective that, their inventors claim, a dieter can reduce some parts of the body, usually the lower parts, while leaving others parts untouched. My experience is that with *all* diets, including the diet advocated here, weight loss is always from the top down. Thus, your chest and then your tummy must lose their excess fat before the excess will start to disappear from your thighs. You cannot do it the other way around.

However, the myth of cellulite has led to a plethora of diets, massage creams and exercises which make their inventors rich but have little effect on the perceived problem.

Liquid protein diets

Most diets allow slimmers to eat 1,000 calories per day. However, a much more worrying trend began when a different form of diet was introduced: the very low calorie liquid protein diets (VLCD). These allowed only between 300 and 600 calories a day. The first was *The Last Chance Diet* devised in 1975 by an osteopath, Robert Linn. His formula was manufactured from sow's belly and cow hide. The resulting 'Prolinn' was a gelatinous protein with little nutritional value and which was so deficient in amino acids as to be insufficient to sustain life. Not surprisingly, there were a number of deaths among those taking it. Although it claimed to affect only body fat, post-mortem examinations on the dieters showed that many who had died had lost a large proportion of protein from their heart muscle.

Although the Last Chance diet was discredited but in 1980, a version of it, *The Cambridge Diet*, was launched, heavily advertised as 'a new scientific breakthrough'. Again a liquid protein diet, the Cambridge Diet was based on skimmed milk. In nutritional terms, this was an improvement on the Prolinn, but not by much. There were more deaths. Other adverse side effects included constipation, diarrhoea, dizziness, headaches, hair loss and loss of blood pressure on rising from a sitting or lying position. In spite of widespread condemnation in the medical press, the Cambridge Diet crossed the Atlantic into Britain in 1985.

In 1983 came the *Amazing Micro Diet*, yet another very-low-calorie liquid diet manufactured by a company trading as Uni-Vite Nutrition. By 1985, its inventors estimated 500,000 Micro-Dieters in Britain. This concoction allowed only 330 calories a day and promised weight losses of between 16 and 20 pounds a month. In their book which explains the diet, the authors show how nutritious it is by comparing it with 330 calories worth of sweets!

These formula diets are real money-spinners. Many of the ingredients which go into their manufacture are waste products of the food industry such as skimmed milk powder and bran. They cost very little but are sold through 'counsellors' at vastly inflated prices. They are dangerous and expensive, yet they sell. History has shown that they are totally unnecessary.

The importance of fat

The science of nutrition is highly complex: nutrients interact so that a deficiency of one can have a profound effect on the metabolism of others. A lack of fat probably causes a wider range of abnormalities than deficiencies of any other single nutrient.

As fat has a high calorific value, all modern low-calorie diets restrict fats. But this can be dangerous and self-defeating. Lack of dietary fat can cause dry skin and eczema, damage to ovaries in females and infertility in males, kidney damage and weight-gain through water-retention in the body. When there is little or no fat in the gut, there is nothing to stimulate the production of bile, the gall bladder is not emptied and the bile is held in reserve. This leads to the formation of gall stones. If a fat-free diet is continued for a long time, the gall bladder may atrophy.

The fat-soluble vitamins A, D, E and K cannot be absorbed from the gut without the presence of fat and bile in the gut. This has consequences for yet more nutrients. Without vitamin D and bile present in the intestine, for example, calcium is not absorbed. For a woman, whose chance of suffering from osteoporosis is high, this is an important consideration. Slimmers are usually told to drink skimmed milk. This has an advantage, they are told, in that it contains more calcium than full-cream milk. This is true – but skimmed milk does not contain very much fat. As a consequence, almost none of the calcium in skimmed milk is absorbed. This small absorption of calcium is reduced still further if the skimmed milk is eaten with a bran-laden breakfast cereal.

All body cells require a continuous supply of various fatty acids. If insufficient are suppied from food, the body tries to make them from sugar. This causes blood-sugar levels to fall, you feel very hungry and eat more, generally of the wrong things – and gain weight.

Fat also has a satiety value: it takes longer to digest and stops you feeling hungry. Eat 100 calories less fat at a meal and you will probably feel hungry so quickly that you will eat three times as many calories in the form of sugary or starchy foods, because they are convenient. Weight gain is inevitable.

Conclusion

The reason that modern slimming diets all fail is because of what they all have in common – they are all low-fat, low-calorie diets that restrict the intake of food to such an extent that the slimmer is starving. The Banting Diet does not restrict calorie intake at all. You really can eat as much as you like provided only that carbohydrate intake is controlled. There are five other important differences, however, and they are:

a. You can live on the Banting diet for the rest of your life without ever again being hungry. There is no stressful 'yo-yo' effect. Instead of starving the weight off, it gets the body to burn fat more efficiently.

b. It is very easy to live with and maintain socially. As all you have to do is reduce your intake of carbohydrates, you can eat what your hostess puts before you without having to disclose that you are 'on a diet'. It is only necessary to take a little more meat and a little less pudding.

c. With this diet, your weight cannot go below your natural weight. This is important. Being overweight may be undesirable but being underweight is potentially far more dangerous as there are serious risks of sudden death associated with extreme leanness.

d. It is a much more healthy diet

e. It is a much more natural diet.

The fifth rule is:
Do not reduce your fat intake.

The major – and most expensive – part of medical technology as applied today appears to be far more for the satisfaction of the health professions than for the benefit of the consumers of health care. Dr Halfdan Mahler, Director General, the World Health Organisation, 1984.

6
THE CHOLESTEROL MYTH

There are several reasons why you might have reservations about taking up any dietary regime that advocates eating fats. The most important is the fear that such a diet is not healthy; that it is the cause of heart disease or cancers.

Over the past decade there has been a growing concern about cholesterol and its role in the aetiology of coronary heart disease. Dieticians, nutritionists and doctors have been telling us that fat is a killer. The British, United States, Australian and Scandinavian governments, among others, have all introduced national policies based around its reduction. Eat less cholesterol, saturated fat and salt, eat more fibre-rich foods we are all told. The evidence is incontrovertible that if we do not, we are doomed to the West's greatest killers – heart disease and cancer.

But is the evidence so clear? Although the public may have been led to believe the propaganda, doctors and scientists have reservations. In the world's medical journals, a great debate is raging: a debate rarely heard by the layman. Is the western diet a killer? Apart from those with a very rare disease, has cholesterol got anything to do with heart disease – or any other disease? And even if it has, will a change of diet be beneficial?

Like all debates, this one about cholesterol has two sides. *The Cholesterol Myth* explores the evidence on which the present 'healthy eating' dietary recommendations are based, concentrating on the side of the debate rarely heard by the non-medical public. The science of nutrition is complex, as is the evidence used in the cholesterol debate. Nevertheless, so much of only one side of the debate has been published and the public has been so brainwashed, that it is necessary to explain the other side in as much detail as this book allows.

58

THE B.M.A. AND THE GOVERNMENT RECOMMEND THAT THE BRITISH PEOPLE SHOULD DRINK 80% MORE MILK, EAT 55% MORE EGGS, 40% MORE BUTTER AND 30% MORE MEAT.

On the basis of research in the 1920s and 1930s by Sir John Boyd Orr and others, that was the advice given to the British people in 1938. The Government introduced free school milk and we 'went to work on an egg'. In consequence, child deaths from diphtheria, measles, scarlet fever and whooping cough fell dramatically – before the introduction of antibiotics and widespread immunisation. Rickets, called 'The English Disease' because it was so widespread, and other deficiency diseases were relegated to the past. Other factors helped, but most important of all was the better nutrition that gave children a higher resistance. The recommendations above shaped our diet for nearly 50 years and helped to give us a mean life-expectancy among the highest in the world. Sixty years in 1930, it climbed to 70 by 1960 and to 75 years by 1990.

Now we are told they are shortening our lives – killing us with coronary heart disease. Why the sudden change? To discover that, we need to know something of the history of coronary heart disease and how the strategy to combat it evolved.

Coronary heart disease

There are various diseases that affect the heart but the one which the 'healthy eating' strategies seek to prevent is Coronary Heart Disease (CHD), otherwise called ischaemic heart disease (IHD). CHD is a condition where the coronary arteries that supply blood to nourish the heart muscle are narrowed by a build-up of material on their walls to such an extent that they become blocked. This cuts off the blood supply to part of the heart muscle, and we have a heart attack. This narrowing also encourages the clotting of blood; and in consequence, it is possible for a clot to cause a heart attack long before the atheroma is large enough to do so. The material generally blamed for the build-up is cholesterol. The 'healthy' eating advice given to the public to reduce the incidence of CHD is aimed simply at reducing the levels of cholesterol in the blood.

Cholesterol. Because of the propaganda, you can be forgiven for thinking that cholesterol is a harmful alien substance which should be avoided at all costs. In fact, nothing could be further from the truth. Cholesterol is an essential component in the body. It is found in all cells, particularly in the brain and nerve cells, and is used to make a number of other important substances such as hormones (including the sex hormones), bile acids and vitamin D. The body uses enormous quantities of cholesterol every day and the substance is so important that every body cell has the ability to make it.

Cholesterol may be ingested in animal products, but less than 20% of the body's cholesterol needs will be supplied in this way. The body then makes up the difference. If less is taken in the diet, the body compensates by making more. Thus the level of blood cholesterol is affected very little by the amount eaten.

Cholesterol and CHD. In 1951, pathologists were sent to Korea to learn about war wounds by dissecting the bodies of dead soldiers. To their surprise they discovered unexpected evidence of coronary heart disease; unexpected for they knew that death from heart disease was extremely rare under the age of 35 and these soldiers averaged only 22 years of age. So, the pathologists performed a detailed dissection on the hearts of the next 300 corpses. In 35% they found deposits of fibrous, fatty material sticking to the artery walls. In a further 41% they found fully formed lesions, and in 3% of the soldiers these lesions were sufficiently large that they blocked at least one coronary artery. Thus, over three-quarters of all the men examined showed evidence of serious coronary heart disease – and they were barely out of their teens.

Doctors now had a problem. As there are no symptoms associated with the partial blockage of the coronary arteries, how could they tell, without a direct examination of those arteries, who was in danger? They had to find what was different in those with the disease and those free from it.

To cut a long story short, they found cholesterol in the material which builds up on artery walls and causes them to become blocked; people who died of heart disease often had high levels of serum cholesterol; and those who suffered the rare hereditary disease, familial hypercholesterolaemia (high blood cholesterol), also suffered more heart attacks. And so, not unnaturally perhaps, cholesterol and CHD became linked.

There are a number of significant points, however, that the cholesterol theory overlooks. For example, there is a marked difference between the build-up found in those with familial hypercholesterolaemia and those with CHD. Hypercholesterolaemia causes large deposits at the mouths of the coronary arteries, often leaving the arteries themselves unblocked, and so does not reproduce the type of obstruction found in coronary heart disease. Also, people with myxoedema or nephrosis have high blood cholesterol levels – yet in them there is no increase in the incidence of CHD. Neither is raised blood cholesterol an indicator of CHD in those over 60. It has also long been known that simple events, such as putting a cuff around the arm prior to taking a sample, or fear of the needle, can result in raised cholesterol values. Even where these are avoided, large fluctuations are known with peak to nadir variations of 15-23%. Lastly, cholesterol is only one of the constituents of an atheroma. If you think about it, cholesterol is so necessary and widespread in the body, that it would have been surprising if it had not been found. Yet the paradox was that the lowering of blood cholesterol became the sole objective in the fight against CHD; and the two principal methods used to achieve this are diet and drugs.

Dietary intervention

The 'diet-heart' strategy has three main pillars. These are:

a. **Eat Less Fat**, particularly saturated fats (mainly from animal products).
b. **Change To Polyunsaturated Fats**. These have been found to lower blood cholesterol levels.
c. **Eat More Fibre.** Fibre is also claimed to lower blood cholesterol.

The eat-less-fat hypothesis was published in 1950 and backed up by Dr Ancel Keys' 'Seven Countries' study in 1953. During the 1970s and early 1980s, results were published of a number of large-scale, long-term, human intervention studies, carried out in many parts of the world which involved hundreds of thousands of subjects and hundreds of doctors and scientists in an attempt to prove that the various elements did indeed reduce the incidence of CHD – and they failed miserably. Not one showed convincing evidence that undertaking a stringent dietary regime had any significant effect on mortality or morbidity from heart disease.

The most influential and respected investigation of the causes of heart disease is the Framingham Study which was begun in 1948. This was the study that gave rise to the 'risk factors' with which we all are so familiar today. The Framingham researchers thought that they knew exactly why some people had more cholesterol than others – they ate more in their diet. To prove the link, they measured cholesterol intake and compared it with blood cholesterol – there was no relationship. Next, they studied intakes of saturated fats – again, there was no relationship; and total calories – yet still there was no relationship to be found. The researchers then considered the possibility that something was masking the effects of diet, but no other factor made the slightest difference.

After 22 years of research, the researchers concluded: 'There is, in short, no suggestion of any relation between diet and the subsequent development of CHD in the study group.'

Table II: *Cholesterol Intake – The Framingham Study*

	Cholesterol Intake mg/day	Blood Cholesterol in Those	
		Below Median Intake mg/dL	Above Median Intake
Men	704 ± 220.9	237	237
Women	492 ± 170.0	245	241

One of the largest and most demanding medical studies ever performed on humans, The Multiple Risk Factor Intervention Trial (MRFIT) involved 28 medical centres and 250 researchers and cost $115,000,000. The researchers screened 361,662 men and deliberately chose subjects who were at very high risk to ensure that they achieved a statistically significant result. They cut cholesterol consumption by 42%, saturated fat consumption by 28% and total calories by 21%. Yet even then they did not succeed. Blood cholesterol levels fell by only a modest amount and, more importantly, coronary heart disease was unaffected. Its originators refer to the results as 'disappointing' and say in their conclusions: 'The overall results do not show a beneficial effect on Coronary Heart Disease or total mortality from this multifactor intervention.'

Table III: *Fat intake and Blood Lipids – The Tecumseh Study*

	Blood Cholesterol in Thirds		
	Lower	Middle	Upper
Daily Intake:			
Fat – total (g)	128	134	133
Fat Saturated (g)	52	54	54
Cholesterol	554	566	533

The Tecumseh Study attempted to correlate blood cholesterol levels measured one day with the amounts of fats eaten the previous day – but found none.

Although not looking for it, the Tecumseh Study also found that blood cholesterol levels were quite independent of whether the dietary fats were saturated or unsaturated. Thus another 'diet-heart' hypothesis, that only saturated fats are to blame, was invalidated.

The results of the World Health Organization European Coronary Prevention Study were called 'depressing' because again no correlation between fats and heart disease was found. They had cut saturated fats down to only 8% of calorie intake daily yet in the UK section there was an increase in heart disease.

North Karelia, which had Finland's highest rates of heart disease was compared with neighbouring Kuopio in The North Karelia Project. In North Karelia, risk factors were cut by 17% over the period of the study and Table IV shows a reduction in both CHD mortality and total mortality. In Kuopio, the control group, however, where there were no restrictions, there was an even bigger decline in CHD and total mortality. These figures suggest that reducing dietary fats, stopping smoking, and so on, may actually have inhibited the decline in heart disease. They certainly offer no support to the diet-heart hypothesis: indeed they suggest that harm was done to those who adopted a 'healthier' lifestyle.

Table IV: *Age Adjusted Rates/1,000. Age Group 30-64 yrs — The North Karelia Project.*

		1970/71	1976/7	Decline
Total Mortality				
Men	N Karelia	13.8	11.6	16%
	Kuopio	13.6	11.4	16%
Women	N Karelia	4.8	3.9	19%
	Kuopio	5.0	3.8	24%
CHD Mortality				
Men	N Karelia	7.7	6.3	18%
	Kuopio	7.7	5.8	25%
Women	N Karelia	2.5	1.7	32%
	Kuopio	2.5	1.6	36%

There is little point in going through the more minor studies; they all show little convincing correlation between either the amount of fat eaten and CHD or the type of fat eaten and CHD. A review of 26 studies published in 1992 concluded that: 'lowering serum cholesterol concentrations does not reduce mortality and is unlikely to prevent coronary heart disease. Claims of the opposite are based on preferential citation of supportive trials.'

Nevertheless, nutritionists and the media continue to mislead the public.

They tell us, for example, that the recent fall in the incidence of heart disease in USA is because Americans are eating less fat. The statistics, however, show clearly that both the rise and fall in CHD coincided with an increase in the amount of fat eaten. While CHD in the USA peaked and started to fall in the 1950s, fat intake rose steadily over the period.

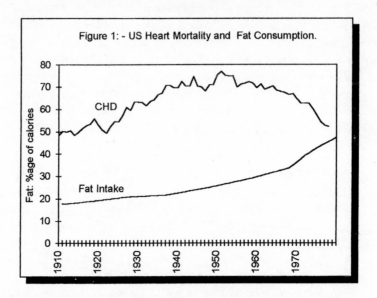

Figure 1: - US Heart Mortality and Fat Consumption.

It is difficult to understand how the fat hypothesis gained such credibility in the USA as their history more than most does not support it. The North American continent had been opened up by explorers and trappers who lived, very healthily, in common with the north American Indians, almost entirely on fresh meat and pemmican. As pemmican is 50% dried lean meat and 50% rendered animal fat, and as fat has over twice the calorific value of protein, they derived over 70% of their calories from fat: that is more than twice the amount currently recommended by dieticians.

We are also told that the British had less CHD in the 1940s when fat was rationed. However, the decade of rationing went on into the early 1950s. The graph at Figure 2 shows clearly that the most rapid rise in CHD occurred during that period.

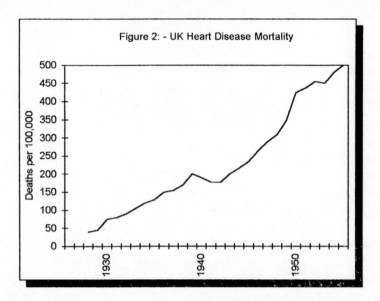

Figure 2: - UK Heart Disease Mortality

Also, during the period of rationing, British farmers had a very low incidence of heart disease – when one would have expected their intake of fats, particularly animal fats, to have been higher than most.

Experience in other countries

The dietary changes in Sweden are similar to those in the USA, yet heart disease mortality in Sweden is rising and American rates are falling. In Japan, intakes of fat have increased by two-thirds since the end of the Second World War. Over the same period their incidence of CHD has fallen consistently. There is also a threefold variation in rates of heart disease between France and Finland even though fat intake in those two countries is very similar. The World Health Organisation is apparently in ignorance of epidemiological data which do not support its recommendation to reduce dietary saturated fat. While it talks of diabetes, hypertension, CHD and cancer being responsible for most deaths in Caribbean countries, fat intake there is remarkably low.

Among South Asians in Britain there is an unusually high incidence of CHD, yet they have lower levels of blood cholesterol and eat diets which are low in saturated fat. Indians in South Africa have probably the highest rates of CHD in the world yet there is no apparent reason why they should based on the current dietary hypotheses. In their own country, south Asian Indians have increased susceptibility to CHD and characteristic lipid abnormalities. Until recently, Indians in India had a remarkably low incidence of CHD using ghee (clarified butter), coconut oil and mustard seed oil – all of which are highly saturated. The epidemic in India of CHD began when these were replaced with peanut, safflower, sunflower, sesame and soyabean oils, all of which are highly polyunsaturated. Indeed, increases in a number of diseases in India are attributed to increased consumption of the essential polyunsaturated fatty acids, linoleic acid and arachidonic acid.

Polyunsaturated fats

The arguments for the polyunsaturated fat hypothesis are no more convincing than those for the cholesterol theory. The claim is that unsaturated fats have a protective or preventative effect on CHD. In Israel, however, when consumption of polyunsaturated fats was about twice that of most Western countries, there was a very high incidence of CHD; the recent decline in the disease in that country followed an increase in the intake of saturated fats. Those given high polyunsaturated diets in a trial in New South Wales fared significantly worse than those on a free diet. And this is the finding in most trials which have increased the ratio of polyunsaturated fats.

From as early as 1971, an excess of cancer deaths has been reported in trials using diets which were high in polyunsaturated fats. In 1991, two studies, from USA and Canada, confirmed independently that the polyunsaturated fatty acid, linoleic acid, enhanced the likelihood of breast tumours. Linoleic acid is the major constituent of all vegetable oils. Polyunsaturated fats are also blamed for a doubling in the incidence of gallstones in the general public.

One of the pioneers of the polyunsaturated-fat-prevents-CHD hypothesis was the American cardiologist E H Ahrens Jr. After twenty-five years of further research, however, he concluded that it was 'irresponsible' to continue to press the polyunsaturated fat recommendations on the general public. He went on:

'If the public's diet is going to be decided by popularity polls and with diminishing regard for the scientific evidence, I fear that future generations will be left in ignorance of the real merits, as well as the possible faults, in any dietary regimen aimed at prevention of coronary heart disease.'

Another of the original proponents of the low-fat, low-cholesterol hypothesis, and a member of the Norwegian Council for Diseases of the Heart and Arteries, Professor Jens Dedichen of Oslo, also changed his mind. In the

1950s Norway had launched a cholesterol-lowering regimen in which soya margarine, which is high in linoleic acid, replaced butter, and soya oil was used extensively. During the subsequent 20 years the increase in the use of soya-based products was accompanied by a steep and continuing rise in deaths from coronary thrombosis. When Dr Dedichen drew attention to the failure of the programme, he received a very hostile reaction from his colleagues.

Also castigated were members of the National Academy of Sciences and the National Research Council of America when, in a report of May 1980, they stated that prevention of heart disease could not be achieved by reduction of blood cholesterol either by diet or drugs, and said that such measures should be abandoned.

Margarine – a natural food?

The polyunsaturated fats used to make margarine are generally obtained from vegetable sources such as rape-seed, cotton-seed and soya bean. As such they might be thought of as 'natural' foods. Usually, however, they are pressed on the public in the form of highly processed margarines, spreads and oils and, as such, they are anything but natural.

In 1989, the petroleum-based solvent, benzene, which is known to cause cancer, was found in Perrier mineral water at a mean concentration of 14 parts per billion. This was enough to cause Perrier to be removed from supermarket shelves. The first process in the manufacture of margarine is the extraction of the oils from the seeds, and this is usually done using similar petroleum-based solvents. These are then boiled off. Nevertheless, this stage of the process still leaves about 10 parts per million of the solvents in the product – that is 700 times as much as 14 parts per billion. The oils then go through more than ten other processes: degumming, bleaching, hydrogenation, neutralization, fractionation, deodorisation, emulsification, interesterification (by this stage, there is hardly any taste left), . . . which include heat treatment at 140-160°F with a solution of caustic soda; the use of nickel as a catalyst, with up to 50 parts per million of the nickel left in the product; the addition of antioxidants such as butylated hydroxyanisole (E320). These antioxidants are usually petroleum-based and are thought by many authorities to be carcinogenic.

The hydrogenation process, which solidifies the oils so that they are spreadable, produces *trans*-unsaturated oils which rarely, if ever, occur in nature. Recent United States studies have shown that heart disease worsened in those who switched from butter to polyunsaturate rich margarine. Research published in March 1993, confirmed this. Women who ate just 4 teaspoons of margarine a day had a 66% *increased* risk of CHD compared to those who ate none. Yet CHD is the one disease which a change to margarine was supposed to reduce!

The heat treatment alone is enough to render these margarines nutritionally inadequate. When the massive chemical treatment and unnatural fats are added, the end product can hardly be called either natural or healthy.

The total amount of fats in our diet today, according to the MAFF National Food Survey, is almost the same as it was at the beginning of this century. What has changed is the types of fats eaten. At the turn of the century, our fat intake was mainly of animal fats, which are largely saturated and mono-unsaturated. Now we are tending to eat more polyunsaturated fats – indeed we are told to. However, two recent studies from the USA and Canada found that linoleic acid, a major constituent of 'high in polyunsaturates' products, is responsible for the rise in the cancers noted in previous studies. Experiments with a variety of fats showed that saturated fats did not cause tumours but, when small amounts of polyunsaturated vegetable oil or linoleic acid itself was added, this greatly increased the promotion of breast cancer.

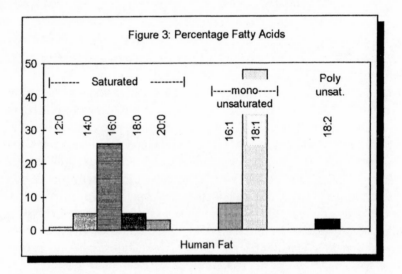

Figure 3: Percentage Fatty Acids

You can see from Figure 3 that the human body's fat make-up is largely saturated and monounsaturated fatty acids. We contain very little polyunsaturated fat.

One of cholesterol's main functions is as a structural part of all body cells.

Cell walls have to allow in the various nutrients from the blood, but stop harmful pathogens. They must be stable. An intake of large quantities of polyunsaturates changes the constituency of cholesterol and body fat. Cell walls become softer and more unstable.

Many laboratories have shown that diets high in polyunsaturates promote tumours. It has been known since at least 1985 that it is linoleic acid which is the major culprit. As Professor Raymond Kearney of Sydney University put it in 1987 'Vegetable oils (eg Corn oil and sunflower oil) which are rich in linoleic acid are potent promoters of tumour growth.'

We are all attacked by carcinogens – background radiation, UV from the sun, particles in the air we breathe and the food we eat. Normally, any small focus of tumour cells is dealt with by the body's immune system and that is the end of it. However, in the presence of a tumour promoter, the tumour may grow too rapidly for the immune system to cope and we get cancer.

Since 1974, the increase of polyunsaturated fats have been blamed for the alarming increase in malignant melanoma (skin cancer) in Australia. We are all told that it is caused by the sun. But Australians are not going out in the sun any more now than they were fifty years ago. However, they are eating more polyunsaturated oils. All victims of the disease have been found to have polyunsaturates in their skin cells. Polyunsaturated oils are oxidised readily by ultra-violet radiation from the sun and form harmful 'free radicals'. These are known to damage the cell's DNA and this can lead to the deregulation we call cancer. Saturated fats do not oxidise and form free radicals.

In this country, you may have heard that malignant melanoma is also on the increase. Is this caused by the sun? It is not likely. In Britain the numbers of sufferers are so small as to be relatively insignificant. Even so, it is not likely that the sun is to blame since the significant increase is in the over-75-year-olds. I cannot imagine that they go out in the sun more. They are eating more polyunsaturated fats, however.

All polyunsaturated margarines, from the brand leader to shops' 'own brands', are around 40% linoleic acid. Butter, on the other hand, has only 2%. Of cooking oils, sunflower oil is 50% and safflower oil 72% while lard has just 9% linoleic acid. We appear to need some linoleic acid for health but the polyunsaturated margarines provide a dangerously high level.

It is interesting to compare the growth of heart disease in this country with intakes of the different fats. Figure 4 plots the birth of CHD in Britain together with the intake of animal fat since the beginning of the century. When these two curves are compared, it is clear that there is no obvious relationship.

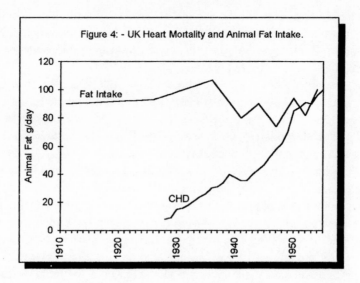

Figure 4: - UK Heart Mortality and Animal Fat Intake.

In Figure 5, CHD is plotted together with intakes of margarines and vegetable shortenings. If there is a causal relationship between fat intake and heart disease, these two graphs suggest to me that it is the margarines and vegetable short- enings which are the more likely candidates for suspicion.

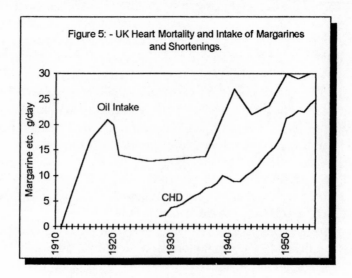

Figure 5: - UK Heart Mortality and Intake of Margarines and Shortenings.

Monounsaturated fats

Several populations in the world, such as Eskimos and those in the Mediterranean countries, eat high-fat diets yet have very low incidences of heart disease. This realisation has led to research scientists switching their attentions to monounsaturated fats such as are found in olive oil.

Although the supposed virtues of monounsaturated fats are being talked of in the press as possible saviours of western man, the monounsaturated theory is not new. It was first demonstrated over thirty years ago that blood cholesterol could be lowered by giving people more unsaturated fats. However, surveys of countries with different tastes in fats and oils have failed to show that this protects against heart disease. For example, Norwegians, who eat a lot of saturated fats have lower rates of the disease than New Zealanders who eat little. But if, as has been suggested, the Norwegians are protected by the mono-unsaturated oils in the fish that they eat, then why is it that in Aberdeen, where a lot of fish is also consumed, the heart disease rate is double that of Oslo? They also forget that there are many other people, such as the Masai tribes of Africa, who eat diets which are low in monounsaturated fats, who also have low incidences of heart disease.

Fibre – the dangerous non-food

The belief that regular bowel movement is important for health is very ancient. But the present theory is based on Dr Dennis Burkitt's discovery that relatively few rural black Africans suffer from cancer of the colon. He attributed this to their relatively crude diet. The theory was that fibre made food travel through the gut faster, thus allowing less time for cancer-inducing agents to form. This, of course, presupposed that food became carcinogenic in the gut and there was no evidence that it did. Neither was there any evidence that moving food through the intestine at a faster rate decreased the risk of colon cancer. Moreover, the rural Africans' lifestyle is far from that of the Western city dweller. Their diet is different, but also they are not exposed to so many pollutants, toxins or mental stresses. Indeed, there are many factors that could be responsible for a difference in disease patterns. Other communities (the Mormons of Utah, for example) also enjoy a low incidence of colon cancer yet eat a low-fibre diet.

So the theory was unsubstantiated at the time and it was to be disproved in practice later as the rural Africans moved into towns and adopted a Western style low fibre diet. Their incidence of colon cancer has remained low and this has continued with the second generation. Nevertheless, these later findings were not publicised. Burkitt's theories caught the attention of the media and, always ready to exploit a good story, they expanded what was at best a very weak hypothesis into a treatment dogma which teaches that fibre is a panacea for all manner of illnesses.

Commercial interests were quick to see the potential in the recommendation. Burkitt's recommendation was based on vegetable fibre, but bran (cereal fibre) has a far higher fibre content and bran was a practically worthless byproduct of the milling process which, until then, had been thrown away. Almost overnight, it became a highly priced profit maker. Although inedible, backed by Burkitt's fibre hypothesis, bran could now be promoted as a valuable food. But Dr Hugh Trowell, another strong advocate of dietary fibre, stated in 1974 that: 'a serious confusion of thought is produced by referring to the dietary fibre hypothesis as the bran hypothesis, for many Africans do not consume cereal or bran '.

Fibre and coronary heart disease. The idea that fibre could protect against CHD was hypothesised by Trowell in 1972, again based on research on rural Africans. The multifactorial intervention trials, however, all concluded that increasing dietary fibre had no effect on CHD.

Fibre and other diseases. Bran has been a popular way to manage irritable bowel syndrome (IBS) for over 20 years, yet several placebo-controlled studies of bran in IBS have shown no convincing beneficial effect. Results from St Bartholomew's Hospital in London, showed clearly that symptoms improved in both placebo and bran groups and there were no significant differences in the two groups' responses. Moreover, there is no direct evidence that an increase of fibre by itself will prevent or cure any of the other diseases. With respect to colon cancer, Burkitt's theory was questioned recently with the suggestion that the low cancer rates in rural Africans may be due to their high early death rates from other causes, so that they do not reach the age at which cancer peaks in Europeans. There is also a growing scepticism in the USA that lack of fibre causes cancer; some studies even suggesting that a fibre-enhanced diet *increased* the risk of colon cancer. Analysis of the data shows that the only significant improvements with bran treatment were in constipation.

But does it matter if we eat fibre? When the supposed benefits of increasing dietary fibre were tested, it soon became apparent that there could be harmful side-effects:

a. All the nutrients in food are absorbed through the gut wall and this takes time. Fibre, by hastening food through the gut faster so that less nutrients are absorbed, inhibits the absorption of iron, calcium, phosphorus, magnesium, energy, proteins, fats and vitamins A, D, E and K.

b. Phytate associated with cereal fibre (bran) also binds with calcium, iron and zinc causing malabsorption. One study, for example, showed that subjects absorbed more iron from white bread than from wholemeal bread even though their intakes of iron were 50% higher with the wholemeal bread.

c. Bran has also been shown to cause faecal losses of calcium, iron, zinc, phosphorus, nitrogen, fats, fatty acids and sterols, thus depleting the body of these materials.

These findings are a cause for concern in several sections of the population who are at considerable risk from eating too much fibre – and bran fibre in particular:

a. The incidence of osteoporosis (brittle bone disease) is increasing and now affects 1 in 2 post-menopausal women, 1 in 5 of whom will die as a direct result. Osteoporosis is caused by several factors, but lack of calcium is the basic problem. Bran both inhibits the absorption of calcium from food and depletes the body of the calcium it has. Moreover, zinc, which bones need to heal, is another mineral whose absorption is adversely affected by cereal fibre.

b. Many sufferers from Alzheimer's Disease (senile dementia) are found to have abnormal amounts of aluminium in their brains. Tests on the people of Guam and parts of New Guinea and Japan, who get Alzheimer's disease at a much younger age, suggest that it is lack of calcium, causing a hormonal imbalance which permits the aluminium to penetrate the brain.

c. Infants may suffer similar brain damage if fed soya-based baby milk as this too has a high phytate content.

d. Vitamin deficiency diseases such as rickets which were common in Britain until a diet high in dairy products and meat was advocated are on the increase again. The situation is getting so bad here that doctors suggest that vegetarian-based fad diets should be regarded as a form of child abuse.

e. In the UK, USA, Canada and South Africa the intake of 'anti-nutrients' such as dietary fibre which impair the absorption of iron, accompanied by a low intake of meat (another result of the diet-heart recommendations), is producing a real risk of iron deficiency anaemia.

f. Depression, anorexia, low birth weight, slow growth, mental retardation, spina bifida and amenorrhoea are associated with deficiencies of zinc and the first five of these are also associated with a deficiency of iron.

g. Lastly, excess fibre affects the onset of menstruation, retards uterine growth and, later, is associated with menstrual dysfunction.

The experts' conclusion is that infants, children, young adolescents, pregnant women and post-menopausal women whose mineral needs are greater should be protected from excessive consumption of fibre.

An assessment of all the cholesterol-lowering dietary trials showed an aggregate 6% *more* deaths in those whose diet had been modified over those on a free diet.

Intervention with drugs

Although it became clear that a change in diet had little effect, that did not end the scientists' efforts to demonstrate that CHD could be prevented. If they could not do it by dietary means, then intervention with drugs would provide the evidence. And since drugs could be controlled much more strictly, and used in conjunction with placebos, the findings would be more demonstrable. But the drugs used to reduce blood cholesterol have all proved to be something of a disaster.

Launched on the public in 1961, **Triparanol** causes the levels of blood cholesterol to fall by inhibiting the liver's ability to make cholesterol. Two years later it was withdrawn because of serious side effects. Luckily for triparanol's manufacturers, a public scandal was avoided as the media's attentions were focused on another drug marketed at the same time and by the same company – thalidomide.

More recently, a number of other drugs have been the subject of extensive and expensive trials. First was **Cholestyramine** (Questran) which reduces cholesterol by interfering with digestion. The gall bladder manufactures bile acid from cholesterol, and the bile acid is used in the intestine to digest fats. But when the drug is present in the gut, it binds with the bile acid, removing it from its normal function. Because the drug is indigestible, it, together with the bile acid, is excreted and the gall bladder has to make more by drawing cholesterol from the bloodstream.

As the trial would be very expensive, the scientists examined 480,000 men over a period of three years to find suitable subjects. They had to be men in the coronary age group and with extremely high blood cholesterol levels. As such men are in the most vulnerable group, their chances of success were greatly increased.

The investigators confidently announced in advance that blood cholesterol levels would be lowered by an average of 28% and, after seven years, coronary heart disease would be reduced by 50% in the treatment group.

At the end of the trial, however, cholesterol levels had fallen by less than a quarter of that called for at the start and heart disease rates were hardly affected. The $142-million trial was a total flop. Even if it had proved a success, however, those participating were so unrepresentative of the population that the question of its efficacy for the typical adult would still have remained. Another flaw that became apparent was an increase in the incidence of oral-gastro-intestinal cancers which could not be dismissed as a random chance. In the Lipid Research Clinics trial there were 21 cases and 8 deaths from gastrointestinal cancer in those taking the drug, compared to 11 cases and 1 death in the control group.

Other organisations tested other drugs. The World Health Organisation sponsored its own trial with **Clofibrate** (Atromid). This too was targeted against cholesterol and was confidently expected to lower blood cholesterol levels by 30%. As with cholestyramine, the levels were lowered by much less than the expected amount and at the end of the trial it became clear that there had been many more deaths in the group taking clofibrate than in the control group – notably from gallstones, cancer of the liver and digestive system. In the WHO clofibrate trial, the drug killed more than it saved.

Among other drugs to be tested were:

a. The female hormone **Oestrogen** on the theory that if pre-menopausal women did not get heart disease, perhaps oestrogen would protect men. But the hormone caused heart attacks rather than preventing them.

b. The hormone **Dextrothyroxine**, which lowers cholesterol levels, was abandoned quickly when an increase in mortality was noticed in the treatment group.

c. The vitamin **Niacin,** which looked promising, but although there appeared to be a reduction in non-fatal heart attacks, there were marked side effects: skin disorders such as darkening, itches and rashes, as well as digestive problems and gout.

d. **Gemfibrozil** (Lopid) was tested and again an increase in deaths was noticed in the treatment group although this time the numbers did not reach statistical significance.

e. **Compactin** which worked in a similar way to triparanol was withdrawn hurriedly and in some secrecy. The reason this time appears to be connected with cancer in dogs.

f. Lastly, despite the previous experiences with triparanol and compactin, yet another inhibitor, **Lovastatin,** has been approved for lifetime use on the general public after tests of very short duration only. (Derivatives pravastatin and simvastatin are marketed as Lipostat and Zocor.)

A study of all trials into cholesterol lowering by drugs up to 1987 showed an *increase* in mortality in those treated with drugs of 13.6%. In 1993 a meta-analysis of all randomised controlled trials of cholesterol-lowering treatments showed that only those with very high risk showed any evidence of benefit. In all others mortality was increased. Its authors conclude that:

> 'Currently evaluated cholesterol-lowering drugs seem to produce mortality benefits in only a small proportion of patients at very high risk of death from coronary heart disease. . . a cautious approach to the use of cholesterol-lowering drugs should be advocated.'

Despite these findings, however, Figure 6 shows that prescriptions rose by nearly eight times in just 6 years!

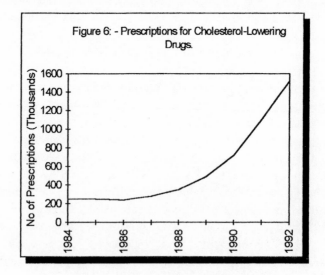

Figure 6: - Prescriptions for Cholesterol-Lowering Drugs.

Low blood cholesterol, cancer and stroke

So far advertisers and news media have concentrated on the supposed danger from high levels of blood cholesterol. The dangers of low blood cholesterol levels have largely been ignored.

Countries with diets high in saturated fats also tend to have high levels of colon cancer. In 1974 a review of the Framingham data and those from Keys' 'Seven Countries' study was carried out. It was expected to show that the cancer could also be blamed on high blood cholesterol. However, the baffled researchers found the opposite: those with the cancer had cholesterol levels which were *lower* than average.

Reports of more than twenty studies into the relation between blood cholesterol and cancer have been published since 1972. Most have reported an association between low blood cholesterol and cancer. The authors of the Renfrew and Paisley Study conclude that 'it may be a mistake to assume that dietary advice given to the general population to reduce the intake of saturated fat will necessarily reduce overall mortality.'

In a study from the USA published in 1990, changes in blood cholesterol over time were studied in patients with colon cancer. The doctors found that there had been an average 13% decline in blood cholesterol levels in the ten years prior to diagnosis of cancer compared with an average increase of 2% in the control group. Both those with the cancer and those free from it had similar blood cholesterol levels initially. It is possible that the decline in blood cholesterol levels was a result of the cancer, not the cause of it, but this is ruled out by the investigators. Comparing studies which reported normal or high cholesterol readings several years prior to diagnosis with others where, at the time of diagnosis, levels were low, they conclude that it was a long term lowering of blood cholesterol levels which gave rise to the cancers. Interestingly, the average blood cholesterol level of those who developed the cancers declined from averages of 6.15 to 5.22 mmol/L in men and 6.8 to 5.9 mmol/L in women, yet the British government's *Health of the Nation* strategy aims to reduce everyone's levels to below 5.2 mmol/L.

More cholesterol but fewer strokes

Published at about the same time was a very-large-scale study in Japan, covering two decades, which concluded that low levels of blood cholesterol also increase the incidence of stroke.

Over the past few decades, Japan has experienced a rapid change in its living and eating patterns. These have resulted in increased consumption of total fat, saturated fatty acids and cholesterol, animal fats and protein, and decreased consumption of carbohydrates (primarily decreased rice consumption). This has provided a unique opportunity for a large-scale, natural experiment into the effects of those changes.

The investigators have shown that the change to Western and urban eating patterns, departing as it does from centuries-old traditions, has caused a general lowering of blood pressure and a large decline in the incidence of stroke deaths and cerebral haemorrhage between the 1960s and the 1980s. They attribute this decline to an increase in blood cholesterol levels over the period. Supporting their findings were the results of a follow-up of 350,000 men screened for the Multiple Risk Factor Intervention Trial in the United States which showed that the excess risk of death from cerebral haemorrhage was raised by 600% in middle-aged men with low blood cholesterol levels.

Low cholesterol and Alzheimer's Disease
Approximately half of the brain is made of fats. Corrigan *et al*, writing in 1991 about the relief of Alzheimer's Disease, ask that 'strategies for increasing the delivery of cholesterol to the brain should be identified'. In the fight against Alzheimer's disease, they recommend *increasing* fat intake.

Has anyone gained?
So far we have been looking at cholesterol-lowering in terms of numbers of deaths, but the trials have had impressive results in the reduction of non-fatal heart attacks and in improvement in the quality of life. Many see this as proof that lowering cholesterol in the total population is a goal worth fighting for.

But those trials were conducted on men rather than on women. They were also conducted on those who had hypercholesterolaemia or, at least, very high blood cholesterol levels – not on people with normal levels. They totally overlook the now well-established non-linear relation between blood cholesterol and heart disease which indicates that lowering blood cholesterol in the general population is not economically worthwhile.

The widespread agreement that the mainstay of the campaign should be a change in diet and lifestyle for all also overlooks the complete lack of evidence that such a course would have any significant effect. It even overlooks the fact that the trials involving cholesterol lowering by dietary means did not show any significant reductions in blood cholesterol.

In 1992 a report of 19 major studies published over the past twenty years suggested that public policy for reducing blood cholesterol should be reviewed. The graph at Figure 7 plots the relative mortality risk from all causes associated with levels of blood cholesterol in men and women. In the case of women, you can see clearly that risk rises as blood cholesterol falls. Dr Hulley states that: 'We are coming to realise that the resulting cardiovascular research, which represents the great majority of the effort so far, may not apply to women'. With men, the situation is more complicated as the curve is U-shaped. However, it still noticeable that low cholesterol is as dangerous as high cholesterol. Dr Hulley concluded that: 'the findings call into question policies built over several decades on evidence that focused only on CHD as an outcome.' He continued: 'it may be time to review national policies aimed at shifting the entire population distribution of blood cholesterol to the left'.

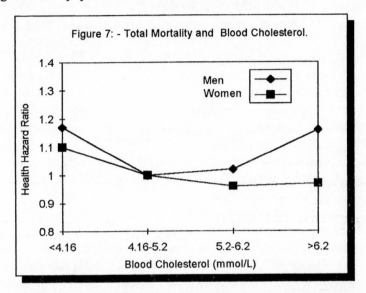

Figure 7: - Total Mortality and Blood Cholesterol.

Another analysis based on a number of American studies has estimated that on a lifelong programme of cholesterol reduction by diet, the gain in life expectancy for those at very high risk (that is the 1 in 500 with hypercholes-terolaemia) would be between 18 days and 12 months, and for those at low risk (that is the other 499) between 3 days and 3 months. That is not very much with which to tempt people to endure a lifetime of unpalatable diets. But these figures assumed that cholesterol lowering was both effective and safe and did not take into account the increased risk of other debilitating and fatal diseases. Once these are added to the equation, it becomes quite evident that the current campaign is virtually certain to do more harm than good. For example, a study of Maoris in New Zealand showed that those with the *lowest* levels of blood cholesterol had the *highest* mortality: findings also borne out by the Framingham Study.

What we have then is a number of very large-scale, long-term, human intervention studies showing that lowering blood cholesterol is possible but that it has no significant beneficial effect on coronary heart disease in the general population, and other studies showing that a low blood cholesterol level, or the methods used to attain it, are increasing the incidence of other serious diseases.

Twenty-five years ago it was said that 'current medical thinking . . . is that while cholesterol may be involved in some way with arteriosclerosis and heart disease, it is no longer held to be the main factor.' and, 'A recent survey of cholesterol findings in geriatric cases involving arteriosclerosis showed a significant number of patients to have normal or low cholesterol.' Those remarks have been confirmed by all the major studies published to date. Forty years after the Framingham Study began, its researchers looked at the question of total mortality and cholesterol. The evidence was that for those with low cholesterol levels, deaths from non-cardiac causes offset any reduced incidence of heart disease. There was 'no increased overall mortality with either high or low serum cholesterol levels' among men over 47 years of age. There was no relationship with women older than 47 or younger than 40. The researchers also concluded that people whose cholesterol levels are falling may be at *increased* risk.

So where does that leave coronary heart disease?
Is coronary heart disease the killer it is made out to be? In 1991 there were nearly 8,000 more deaths attributed to CHD than in 1971, but an analysis of the figures shows that all of that increase is in those over 70 years of age.

Table V: *CHD Mortality in UK Over Age 70 by Sex and Age*

Ages	70-74	75-79	80-84	Over 85
Men				
1971	13609	11334	7928	5886
1991	13930	15472	12672	9368
Women				
1971	9762	11928	11550	12749
1991	8586	12633	15301	21134

ICD 410-414

If we look at what might appear to be the worst case – women over 85 – there has been an increase of almost 70%. But does this illustrate a problem? No. It is a fallacy to believe that if these people had modified their diet or lifestyle, they would still be alive. We are not an immortal species and cannot expect to live forever. The figures merely show that more women survived to an age greater than 85 years in 1991 than did in 1971. The same is true of all ages and both sexes and that, surely, is a good thing.

This increase in longevity is confirmed if we look at the figures for CHD deaths in those under 70. Table VI illustrates clearly that CHD rates have fallen considerably in all age groups and both sexes over the past two decades. Mortality in men under 65 has fallen by 40% over the period.

Table VI: *CHD Mortality in UK Under Age 70 by Sex and Age*

Ages	40-44	45-49	50-54	55-59	60-64	65-69
Men						
1971	1436	3153	4900	7850	11608	14603
1991	862	1527	2766	4616	7886	12064
Women						
1971	201	467	933	1870	3845	6657
1991	144	262	538	1273	2855	5666

ICD 410-414

And do not be misled into believing that this reduction is as a result of the 'healthy eating' recommendations; they are much too recent and insufficiently widespread to have had such a marked impact. The people in the later groups are those who were brought up or who spent the greater part of their lives with the recommendations with which this chapter began. These people had free, full cream milk at school and ate such food as bread and dripping. During the period after World War II when deaths from CHD levelled off and started to fall, a diet which was relatively high in fat was the vogue.

Not that this will come as any surprise to the Medical Research Council. In its report on the Caerphilly Study published in 1993, the MRC's Epidemiology Unit at Cardiff showed that men who drank more than a pint of full-cream milk a day had only one-tenth the incidence of heart disease as those who drank none. They also demonstrated that those who ate a high-energy diet lived longer than those who cut dietary fats. Their findings indicate that far from being a killer, the diet we are told to avoid by the nutritionists may actually be protective against heart disease!

Fat has over twice the energy value of either carbohydrates or proteins, and other essential nutrients such as: lipids used in the brain and central nervous system without which we become irritable and aggressive; sterols, precursors of the bile acids and a number of hormones (including the sex hormones); and the fat-soluble vitamins A, D, E and K. Fat has been called 'the most valuable food known to man'. It is both stupid and wasteful to throw it away.

The Mediterranean diet

The Mediterranean diet is healthier than ours, we are told. We should eat what the French, Italians and Spanish eat. This observation is based on the fact that the peoples of the southern part of Europe appear to suffer a lower incidence of heart disease. Again, simplistically, this is attributed entirely to a difference in diets. Other factors which might have an effect are ignored. For example, it is noticeable that CHD rates increase as one travels north. It could be the weather! In Scotland, the incidence of the disease is greater in the west than in the east. The only real difference between the two is that it rains more in the west. It is unlikely that there is much difference in their relative diets. However, since they comparing European and British diets, let us do just that.

The 'Mediterranean' diet is what the health fanatics advocate because, they say, it is low in fat. Obviously, they have never been there. They don't seem to know that northern Italians eat butter. They have not noticed that the Spanish spread pork dripping thickly on toast for breakfast. And nobody has told them that goose fat is used to make *cassoulet* in the south of France or that, throughout the Mediterranean, the sausages, salamis and pâtés are all up to 50% fat. The Mediterranean diet may be healthier but, contrary to popular belief, it is a *high*-fat diet! Indeed, the Mediterranean diet is considerably higher in fat than the British 'healthy eating' diet.

However, there are a number of major differences in dietary practices between Britain and the Mediterranean countries which may play a significant part in their effects on health. Not only is the food which is eaten by the average working family in southern Europe very different from that eaten by a typical family in Britain, more importantly perhaps, the way it is bought, presented and eaten is also different. A brief list of the principal differences is tabled below.

Mediterranean Eating Pattern	British Eating Pattern
The average Mediterranean diet comprises natural, unprocessed meat, vegetables and fruit, which are usually bought fresh daily.	The average British diet is composed of packaged, highly processed foods with chemical additives.
Meat plays an important part.	We are told to eat less meat.
Fats eaten are butter, olive oil and unprocessed animal fats.	Fats eaten are highly processed margarines, low-fat butter substitutes, and vegetable oils.
Meals are taken slowly, without hurrying. Lunch usually takes up to two hours – and is followed by a siesta.	In Britain, food is rushed. Lunches are eaten on the run or combined with work. Often, they are junk-food snacks.
Wine (believed to be protective against heart disease), is drunk during meals as part of that meal.	Beer, wines and spirits are drunk in the evening after the evening meal.
Most of the day's energy intake is eaten before 2.00 pm	The biggest meal is at the end of the day.

Cholesterol testing

A last thought, if you are still thinking of having your cholesterol tested. Imagine it's 2.00 am and you are lying in bed. You hear a noise downstairs which you know is caused by a burglar. You know how quickly your heart starts to race. Well that is how quickly your cholesterol level can rise – and for the same reason. For raised blood cholesterol is part of the 'fight-or-flight' reflex. If, when you visit your doctor, you have been running, your cholesterol level will be higher that if you walked. If you have been standing, it will be higher than if you've been sitting. If you are anxious or the doctor looks worried it will be higher. And, if you go to the surgery, it will be higher than if the test is done at home. If blood cholesterol were tested hourly throughout a day, or daily over a month, it would not be unusual to find a wide variation in values. It also rises naturally as you get older so that while a reading of 9 mmol/L is high at 20, it is not abnormal if you are 50.

Cholesterol measurements are not very accurate (less than 80%) even when conducted in a laboratory. A survey showed that on the same sample, laboratories could differ by as much as 1.3 mmol/L. When done in a doctor's desktop machine the accuracy will inevitably be lower.

To put it in perspective, let us assume that you are around 30 years old and your cholesterol level is a respectable 6.0 mmol/l. You run to the surgery and are anxious about the result. This could raise it by 25% to 7.5. It is sent to a laboratory giving the high readings and it is raised by a further 1.3. Your perfectly normal 6.0 is now a high 8.8!

The fact is that so many variables affect cholesterol levels that a one-off test is a waste of time. It is an unnecessary worry which can do more harm than good. Bear that in mind if you are subjected to a cholesterol test.

Conclusion
More resources, time and money have been spent over the last forty years on CHD than any other disease in medical history and all it has proved is that doctors don't know as much as they thought they did. If over forty years of serious research has failed to find a causal link between the various risk factors and CHD, it can only be because there is no link. The biggest crusade in medical history is based on hypotheses and recommendations supported only by inconclusive evidence and wildly inaccurate measurements.

Preventative measures are becoming compulsory – in the USA, people can be refused medical and life insurance if they do not abide by the recommendations – and the rights of consent and personal freedom are being lost. These important decisions are being made on the outcome of unreliable tests.

If you are to make intelligent decisions and take up healthy eating practices, you must be given advice which is based on fact rather than unfounded assumptions. And the facts seem to be that full-cream milk, cream, butter, meat and fresh fruit and vegetables are the healthy foods whilst 'high-in-poly-unsaturates' spreads and oils, wholemeal bread, bran flakes and packaged foods are not. If we consider our evolutionary past, this is not really surprising.

There is no evidence of a need to endure an unpalatable fatless, bran-laden diet. Apart from being less pleasurable to eat, the evidence is clear – 'healthy eating' is not so healthy after all.

A food is not necessarily essential just because your child hates it. Katherine Whitehorn

7

OTHER MYTHS DISPELLED

Banting's diet is such that so long as carbohydrate intake is reduced, there is no restriction on the amount of food you can eat. That should be enough to stop anyone objecting to it. However, no doubt someone will. Below are some possible objections and their answers.

There are several arguments that may be used against this diet. The objections that a high-fat diet is fattening, or will lead to heart disease have already been refuted. This chapter will cover the rest.

The balanced diet

There is no concept so dear to a nutritionist's heart as that of a balanced diet and it will undoubtedly be said by some that the type of diet advocated by Banting is not a balanced diet. To tell us what our balanced eating patterns should be, tables are published in most countries which divide food into groups. We are told that if we are to remain healthy, we must include food from each of these groups in our diets. Tables vary from country to country, but they are basically the same. Table VII is a typical example of its type.

You will realise just how necessary a 'balanced' diet is when you consider that in many parts of the world large groups of hunters live quite healthily on nothing but a small part of the first group. It must be obvious from the evidence presented so far that men can and do remain fit on diets which are restricted to meat alone. And that observation is not confined to those one might call primitives – the Eskimo and Masai for example. Apart from Stefansson and Anderson, the gauchos of Argentina, mainly descendants of European settlers, are near to being pure carnivores, as they live healthily almost exclusively on beef. Obviously, the 'balanced' diet so beloved of dieticians is not so important after all.

Table VII. *A Typical 'Balanced Diet' Table*

Eat some food from each group every day
Meat, poultry, fish and eggs or dried beans, peas and nuts.
Milk and milk products.
Butter or margarine fortified with vitamins A and D.
Bread, flour and cereals.
Green and yellow vegetables.
Potatoes and other vegetables.
Fruits such as oranges, grapefruit and tomatoes.

The truth is that a balanced diet is any diet which supplies all the nutrients the body requires, in the proportions it requires. A diet of fresh meat alone can do just that. Banting's diet, however, goes much further in that carbohydrate intake is not banned, merely reduced. It is, in all respects, a balanced diet.

A high-fat diet is nauseous

Some may object, saying that they find a high-fat diet nauseous. They associate the word 'fat' with blubber or greasy food. It is noticeable, however, that they usually have no difficulty eating fat if it is called butter or cream, or served to them in bacon or in a suet pudding. The person who cannot stand 'greasy food' usually has no problem with chocolate.

Strangely, although people have been professing to want leaner meat since the end of food rationing in the 1950s, the actual consumption of fat both in Britain and in the USA has been rising steadily throughout the 20th century.

If you really cannot stand the sight of visible fat on a succulent piece of meat, however, you can avoid offending your palate by choosing foods which are high in invisible fats or the acceptable fats which you eat now. After a while you will find that you will come to relish the crackling on pork or fat on a piece of roast beef and you will be back to the ideal diet.

Ketosis

There is another objection which may be brought up by your physician and which must be addressed. This is that high-fat diets may cause an undesirable condition called ketosis. Ketones are a class of compounds which are quite normal products of fat metabolism. They can be oxidised in the body to provide a source of energy. However, elevated levels of ketones can occur when there is an imbalance in fat metabolism. This condition is called ketosis. People unable to use glucose as an energy source, such as diabetics, tend to suffer from this condition. It is also found in people who are starving.

In the case of diabetes, the level of ketones is very high, often over 300 mg per 100 ml. The levels of ketones in the blood of someone on the Banting diet is insignificant compared to this; even lower in fact than in a person who is fasting or on a low-calorie diet. In the clinical trials of the Banting high-fat, low-carbohydrate diet, ketosis was never a problem. While there are clearly various levels of ketosis, they all have a common cause: dietary deficiencies of carbohydrate. There was a catch phrase for medical students that 'fat burns only in the flame of carbohydrates'. A *Family Doctor* booklet entitled *Feeding The Family* published by the B.M.A. said:

'Fat is burned down by the body to carbon and water, but to do this, there must be carbohydrates present. Otherwise, the breakdown is not complete and what are called ketone bodies pass into the blood and urine. This causes sweetish breath and biliousness.'

Anyone who has studied nutrition will view this statement with some scepticism. History tells us that man, in many parts of the world, has lived, indeed still does live, healthily on dietary regimes which exclude all carbohydrates except the small amount that is found in meat. The 60 grams a day which are included in the dietary regime advocated here, should be more than enough to allay any fears.

Sweet cravings

The last objections may be concerned with the overweight person's craving for sweet things and with cost. Carbohydrate foods such as potato crisps, chocolate or bread and jam tend to be more readily available for snacks than meat and cheese. It is easier, therefore, for a person to over-eat sweet, carbohydrate-rich foods. This is particularly true where the person is eating what he is used to, and where well-meaning friends press such food on him. Sweet and starchy foods are also cheaper to buy. But anyone prepared to spend good money on dubious slimming clubs and magazines, would be better advised to spend that money on good wholesome food. It need not cost more than the membership fees. And by eating properly, there will be no need to snack on sweets.

And ye shall live off the fat of the land. Genesis 45, 18.

8
BANTING IN PRACTICE

The Banting low-carbohydrate diet is very simple in concept. You can eat as much as you want of any meat, fish, poultry, cheese, cream, butter – in fact all the things which are high in proteins and fats. Although there are some carbohydrate foods, such as sugar, which it may be advisable to cut out altogether, it is not necessary to stop eating fruit, vegetables and cereals: merely cut down. For maximum weight-loss, it is necessary only to reduce your intake of them so that it is about 60 grams per day. Note, however, that the 60-gram limit is only a starting point while you are slimming. Once you are down to your correct weight, it will be possible to increase your intake without regaining weight. It is also possible that you will achieve a weight loss, albeit more slowly, merely by reducing your intake of the more carbohydrate-dense foods such as those listed below.

The foods which have the densest carbohydrate content, and which you should be most wary of, while you are overweight, are:

Bread and biscuits.
Rice and pasta.
Cakes, sweet pies, puddings and other sweet desserts.
Jams, jellies, honey, syrups and sugar.
Sweet, fizzy drinks, unless they are low-calorie.
Beer and sweet wines.
Fruits which are tinned or cooked in syrup.
Dried fruits.

You do not have to go through life never tasting these again. They are mentioned because they are the foods with the highest carbohydrate content.

As you get used to managing this diet you can re-introduce them. At Appendix B is a full list of common foods and their carbohydrate contents.

There is one other caveat; milk is fairly high in carbohydrate. It should be restricted to about half a pint per day. If you prefer tea or coffee with milk, try using cream instead.

Some weight watchers have difficulty giving up certain foods. Bread seems to prove a particular problem but you do not have to give up eating bread altogether. Just cut down or substitute a starch-reduced bread. If you like juice at breakfast, drink grapefruit in preference to orange and reduce the amount. Breakfast could be, for example, grapefruit juice, fried egg and bacon, a slice of thickly buttered toast and coffee with cream and a non-sugar sweetener. You are off to a good start for the day, yet you have only eaten about 18 grams of carbohydrate. Compare this with a small bowl of cornflakes and a quarter of a pint of skimmed milk which would be about 30 grams of carbohydrate. That is half your daily carbohydrate allowance and you have hardly eaten anything.

The importance of breakfast

Slimmers are usually recommended to take meals spread out over the day, rather than have one large one, and that the pattern should be 'breakfast like a king, lunch like a lord and dine like a pauper'. In other words, the biggest meal should be at the start of the day, when energy for work is required, instead of the more usual practice of having it in the evening when all one is going to do is sit and watch television and go to bed. This makes sense. Several lines of research have suggested that both children and adults get fatter and do not perform as well if they do not have breakfast. The average working person needs some 2,500 or more calories a day. If he is to spread his calorie intake out over the day sensibly, he must think in terms of eating a breakfast of up to, say, 800 to 1,000 calories. And this cannot be achieved on muesli and skimmed milk.

Breakfast is important, it determines what your blood-sugar levels will be throughout the day. The constituents of your breakfast are also important. Both how much you eat and what you eat for breakfast determine how you will feel and act, and how efficiently you will operate. Eating too much of the wrong foods is as bad as not eating enough of the right ones.

Many studies have been conducted into the effects of various foods at breakfast time. In one, subjects ate a variety of typical breakfasts. To assess their relative influence, blood sugar levels were measured before breakfast and then at hourly intervals for three hours afterwards.

The findings, looked at today, are quite remarkable. The breakfasts that are the most popular today are the ones that gave the worst results in the tests:

a. Black coffee alone caused a drop in blood-sugar levels, and feelings of hunger, fatigue, lassitude, irritability, nervousness, exhaustion and headaches, which got progressively worse.

b. Two doughnuts and coffee with cream and sugar caused a rapid rise in blood-sugar, which fell within one hour to a low level giving similar symptoms to the coffee-only breakfast.

c. The typical American breakfast of: a glass of orange juice, two strips of bacon, toast, jam and coffee with cream and sugar was tested. Again, blood-sugar rose rapidly but fell to a level far below the pre-breakfast level within an hour, remaining low until lunchtime.

d. The fourth breakfast was the same as the last except that it had breakfast cereal added. The result was the same: a rapid rise followed quickly by a fall to abnormally low levels.

e. The fifth breakfast was again the typical breakfast except that the cereal was replaced with oatmeal served with milk and sugar. Again there was a rapid rise in blood-sugar followed by a fall which, this time, was more rapid and to an even lower level.

f. Lastly, the typical breakfast of orange juice, bacon, toast, jam and coffee was served with two eggs. This time, blood-sugar levels rose and stayed up all morning, as did efficiency and a feeling of well-being. A similar breakfast, replacing the eggs with fortified full-cream milk was also beneficial.

The effects of the various breakfasts on the subjects were then studied after they had eaten lunch. Those who had eaten the most protein at breakfast, retained a high blood-sugar level all afternoon. When blood-sugar levels had been low in the morning, after the largely carbohydrate breakfasts, however, levels after lunch rose only for a matter of minutes, falling to a low level which lasted all afternoon. The amount of protein at breakfast time is highly relevant.

Since then, several similar studies have been conducted. The results have been consistent: efficiency and a feeling of well-being experienced after meals is directly related to the amount of protein eaten. Twenty-two grams of protein were required for a breakfast to be effective but the best results were obtained then breakfast contained 55 grams. To put those figures in perspective, an egg contains about 6 grams and an average slice of bacon, 4 grams of protein. The best breakfasts of all were those which also included fat and a little carbohydrate. This was true of all meals.

There are other advantages to taking a breakfast, whatever its size. Breakfast, for most people, is followed by a trip to the lavatory. This is caused by the 'gastrocolic reflex' which works best in the morning. Although a cup of coffee can set off this reflex action, the strongest stimulus is dietary fat. That may be another good reason for a breakfast of eggs and bacon. Anyone who is constipated would do well to cultivate the breakfast habit.

From a slimming point of view, other studies have shown that fat children eat smaller breakfasts and have bigger dinners than their leaner playmates. This evidence confirms that, in the effort to slim, large breakfasts and small dinners should be the order of the day. There can be no doubt that breakfast is the most important meal of the day. Miss other meals if you must, but never miss breakfast.

The diet

It is as well to be aware of what you are trying to achieve before starting this diet. What you are embarking on is an unrestricted-calorie diet; a diet which is probably like no other diet you have ever tried. You may be eating between 2,000 and 3,000 calories a day. But don't bother counting them, they are irrelevant. You are, however, going to restrict your intake of sweet and starchy foods. You may find that merely cutting down on them is sufficient, or you may have to make a more conscious effort to avoid eating too much of them. Let your appetite be your guide, eat as much protein and fat as you need. Historically people have preferred them one part fat to three parts lean.

Remember the first rule: **if you are not overweight, don't diet**. If you are within the acceptable weight-range for your height, you may not lose any weight on this diet. (If you are within the acceptable weight-range for your height, there is no reason why you should not adopt the diet's principles as a precautionary measure. That should ensure that you never do become overweight.)

It is dangerous to lose weight too quickly, particularly if you are only moderately overweight. **You should never try to lose more than 2 lbs per week.** You may find that you do lose more than that in the first week or so. This is normal on any new diet.

Using the tables of carbohydrate content at Appendix B, start by restricting your daily intake to 60 grams a day and see how your weight changes. Sixty grams is only a starting point – you may be lucky and find that you can eat more. **You should not cut your carbohydrate intake to below 60 grams.** Note that this regime will not let your weight go below your natural weight. If your weight is already within the acceptable range and you want to be skinny, this diet won't work. That is one reason why it is so much healthier than low-calorie diets. They rely on starvation to achieve results.

Remember, fat is slimming and fat is healthy. Do not cut fat off meat. Do not remove the skin from chicken, duck or turkey. Do not use skimmed milk.

There are some suggested menus at Appendix C, but below is a broad pattern your meals for the day should follow:

Breakfast. Have a good old-fashioned breakfast of a selection of: fried bacon, eggs, kidneys, omelettes; cold meats, ham and continental sausage (British sausage, unfortunately, usually has a high proportion of cereal filler and is high in carbohydrates); kippers, bloaters, haddock either fried or stewed in milk and butter; tea or coffee with a little milk or plenty of cream, artificial sweetener if required but no sugar; starch-reduced bread with butter or peanut butter but not jam or marmalade.

After such a breakfast you should not get hungry and you should not need to eat anything until lunchtime, but you should drink at least three cups of liquid: tea or coffee with cream and artificial sweetener, or water.

Lunch. For lunch you may eat any meat with its fat left on; fish, poached, grilled or fried (not in batter); cold meats; omelettes; cheese with salad or a serving of green vegetables with as much butter as you like. An apple or other small fruit, cheese, coffee or tea with cream or a little milk but no sugar.

Dinner. Dinner follows the same rules as breakfast and lunch. If you like an alcoholic drink with your meal, bear in mind its carbohydrate content and treat it as any other food. Dry drinks are recommended.

If after all that you do feel the need to nibble something, have a piece of cheese, an ounce of peanuts or a hard-boiled egg.

Incidentally, some years ago I had a job which required me to take my lunch with me. In this situation most people take sandwiches, but sandwiches are made with bread, and bread is high in carbohydrates. I did take sand-wiches, however, in the form of two slices of processed cheese, buttered and with a slice of meat in the middle. It was a bit too rich and I did not keep it up for long but it does show what can be done. Now, in this situation I would take a covered bowl of salad, or meat, cheese and pickles.

When you have reached the acceptable weight for your height and age, you may increase the amount of carbohydrate in your diet or indulge yourself on chocolate once a week. But watch the scales occasionally and if your weight starts to creep up, just reduce your intake of the carbohydrates again.

Aids to dieting

To help you to stay with a diet, it is a good idea not to have foods in the house to tempt you. You cannot have biscuits with your mid-morning cup of tea, if there are none in the biscuit barrel. When you shop, make a list and stick to it. If you are going to treat yourself to a bar of chocolate at the weekend, don't buy it on the previous Monday – you might be tempted to eat it sooner than you planned. Your weight will fluctuate from day to day (indeed it will fluctuate throughout the day), and for women, throughout the month. Resist the temptation to weigh yourself daily. Once a week is quite sufficient. When you do weigh yourself, do it on the same day, at the same time, and in the same clothes (or, preferably, no clothes) each time.

This dietary regime may be new to you but it is one which has proven itself for nearly one and a half centuries. It is completely safe and may be eaten for life. No other diet offers so much. In fact it offers so many filling foods to satisfy you that the small sacrifice you make by reducing your carbohydrate intake is really no sacrifice at all. You need never be hungry again. And this diet really does work.

So try it – what have you got to lose?

APPENDIX A
ADULT HEIGHT/WEIGHT TABLES

In the following tables, heights are measured without shoes and weights without clothes. If indoor clothing is worn, their weight should be added. Estimated weights of indoor clothing are: 7-9 lbs for men and 4-6 lbs for women.

Imperial Height And Weight Tables For Men And Women Ages 25-59 years

Height	Men Weight Range (lbs)		Women Weight Range (lbs)	
Ft Ins	Acceptable	Obese	Acceptable	Obese
4 9			99 - 128	154
4 10			100 - 131	157
4 11			101 - 134	161
5 0			103 - 137	164
5 1	123 - 145	174	105 - 140	168
5 2	125 - 148	178	108 - 144	173
5 3	127 - 151	181	111 - 148	178
5 4	129 - 155	186	114 - 152	182
5 5	131 - 159	191	117 - 156	187
5 6	133 - 163	196	120 - 160	192
5 7	135 - 167	200	123 - 164	197
5 8	137 - 171	205	126 - 167	200
5 9	139 - 175	210	129 - 170	204
5 10	141 - 179	215	132 - 173	208
5 11	144 - 183	220	135 - 176	211
6 0	147 - 187	224		
6 1	150 - 192	230		
6 2	153 - 197	236		
6 3	157 - 202	242		

APPENDIX A 95

Metric Height And Weight Tables For Men And Women
Ages 25-59 years

Height	Men Weight Range (kg)		Women Weight Range (kg)	
m	Acceptable	Obese	Acceptable	Obese
1.45			50.8 - 58.0	69.9
1.47			45.4 - 59.5	71.2
1.49			46.0 - 60.5	73.0
1.52	55.5 - 65.5	79.0	47.5 - 63.5	76.0
1.55	56.5 - 67.0	80.5	49.0 - 65.5	78.5
1.57	57.5 - 68.5	82.0	50.5 - 67.0	80.5
1.60	58.5 - 70.0	84.5	51.5 - 69.0	82.5
1.62	59.5 - 72.0	86.5	53.0 - 70.5	85.0
1.65	60.5 - 74.0	89.0	54.5 - 72.5	87.0
1.67	57.5 - 75.5	90.5	55.5 - 74.0	89.5
1.70	62.0 - 77.5	93.0	57.0 - 75.5	90.5
1.72	63.0 - 79.5	95.5	58.5 - 77.0	92.5
1.75	64.0 - 81.0	97.5	60.0 - 78.5	94.5
1.77	65.5 - 83.0	100.0	61.0 - 80.0	95.5
1.82	66.5 - 85.0	101.5		
1.85	68.0 - 87.0	104.5		
1.87	69.5 - 89.5	107.0		
1.90	71.0 - 91.5	109.5		

Prepared from data published by the Metropolitan Life Insurance Company 1983.

APPENDIX B
CARBOHYDRATE CONTENT OF FOODS

This appendix contains two tables. The first gives the carbohydrate content of common foods in normal servings. The second table gives carbohydrate contents for a wider range of foods in grams per 100 grams (3½ oz).

Carbohydrate contents of common foods

For easy reference, below is a list of the carbohydrate content (in grams) of common foods. As all foods from animals, fish and birds are low in carbohydrate and may be eaten freely, these are not included. Only foods of vegetable origin, and only then those which have a relatively concentrated carbohydrate content, need be avoided.

Food	Carbohydrate	Food	Carbohydrate
Fruit		Nectarine, raw, 5oz	16
Apple, small	10	Orange, 3" diam	9
medium	13	Orange juice, ½ pint	24
large	21	Peach, 2" diam	9
Apricot, raw	2	Pear, medium	14
dried	10	Pineapple, raw, 1oz	3
Banana, small	15	Plums, raw, 4oz	10
medium	16	Prunes, dried, with stones	9
Blackberries, raw, 1 oz	2	Raspberries, raw, 1oz	2
Cherries, raw, 1oz	40	Rhubarb, stewed,	
Clementine	5	no sugar, 5oz	1
Currants, dried, 1oz	18	Strawberries, raw, 1oz	2
Damsons, raw, 1oz	2		
Dates, dried, 1oz	18	**Nuts**	
Fig, raw, one	4	Almonds, 1oz	1
Gooseberries, raw, 1oz	1	Brazils, 1oz	1
Grapefruit, raw, 7oz	5	Cashews, roast, 4oz packet	18
juice, unsweetened, ½ pint	20	Chestnuts, shelled, 1oz	10
Grapes, 1oz	4	Cobs, 1oz	2
Melon, raw, 6oz	5	Coconut, raw, 1oz	1

Food	Carbohydrate	Food	Carbohydrate
Coconut, dessicated, 1oz	2	Muffin (1)	28
Hazelnuts, 1oz	2	Roll (1)	30
Peanuts, roasted, 1oz	2	Flour, plain, 1oz	23
Walnuts, raw, 1oz	1	Oats, raw, 1oz	21
		Pasta, (all types), dry 1oz	7
Cereals		Pasta verde, dry, 1oz	22
Breakfast cereals, see below		cooked, 1oz	6
Butter biscuit, (2)	15	Pastry, 1oz	10-14
Cream cracker (4)	19	Porage, made with	
Digestive (2)	19	water, 4oz	9
		Rice, white, raw, 1oz	25
Water biscuit (4)	21	boiled, 1oz	8
Bread, slice, small	12	Sugar, 1oz	30
Croissant (1)	30	Honey, 1oz	22
Crumpet (1)	16		

The carbohydrate content of breakfast cereals is marked on their packets.

Vegetables
Most green vegetables are low in carbohydrate and are not listed. It is the root vegetables and seeds which tend to have a relatively high carbohydrate content. They are listed below. As a rough guide, restrict yourself to about a cup of vegetables (measured after cooking) per meal. Greens may be eaten in larger quantities.

Food	Carbohydrate	Food	Carbohydrate
Beans, baked, 2tbs	4	Corn on the cob, raw, 5"	34
broad, raw, 1oz	2	Lentils, dried, 1oz	15
butter, dried, 1oz	14	Onion, medium	3
french, raw, 1oz	0	Parsnips, raw, 1oz	3
haricot, dried, 1oz	13	Peas, raw, 1oz	3
runner, raw, 1oz	1	Potatoes, raw, 4oz	24
Beetroot, raw, medium	6	Sweetcorn, canned, 1oz	5
Carrots, raw, 4oz	5	Turnips, raw, 1oz	1

Carbohydrate content of foods in grams per 100 grams

Food	Carbohydrate	Food	Carbohydrate
Milk		**Fish**	
Cream - single	3	White fish	0
Milk, liquid, whole	5	Cod, fried	7
liquid, skimmed	5	Fish fingers	16
dried, skimmed	50	Herrings	0
Yoghurt, low-fat, natural	10	Mackerel	0
low-fat, fruit	18	Pilchards, canned in tomato sauce	1
		Prawns, boiled	0
Cheese		Sardines, canned in oil, fish only	0
Cheddar	0	Tuna in oil	0
Cottage	1		
Cheese spread	1	**Eggs**	
Feta	0	Eggs, boiled or fried	0
Brie	0		
		Fats	
Meat		Lard, cooking fat, dripping	0
Bacon, rashers	0	Margarine, average	0
Beef, mince, stewed	0	Cooking and salad oil	0
stewing steak	0		
Black pudding, fried	15	**Preserves, etc.**	
Chicken, roast, meat and skin	0	Chocolate, milk	59
Corned beef	0	Honey	76
Ham	0	Jam	69
Kidney, pig's, fried	0	Marmalade	70
Lamb, roast	0	Sugar, white	100
Liver, lamb's, fried	0	Syrup	79
Luncheon meat	3	Peppermints	100
Pâté, average	1		
Pork chop, cooked	0	**Vegetables**	
Sausage, beef, cooked	15	Aubergines	3
pork, cooked	11	Baked Beans	15
Steak & kidney pie	22	Beans, runner, boiled	3
Turkey, roast, meat and skin	0	Beans red kidney, raw	45

Food	Carbohydrate	Food	Carbohydrate
Beans, soya, boiled	9	Avocado pear	2
Beetroot, boiled	10	Bananas	19
Brussels sprouts, boiled	2	Blackberries, raw	7
Cabbage, raw	3	Blackcurrants	7
boiled	2	Cherries	12
Carrots, old	5	Clementine	8
Cauliflower, cooked	1	Cranberries, raw	4
Celery	1	Currants, dried	59
Courgettes, raw	5	Dates, dried	64
Cucumber	2	Figs, dried	53
Lentils, cooked	17	Gooseberries, raw	4
Lettuce	1	cooked, unsweetened	3
Mushrooms	0	Grapes	16
Onion	5	Grapefruit	5
Parsnips, cooked	14	Lemon juice	2
Peas, frozen, boiled	11	Mango	15
Peas canned, processed	19	Melon, raw	4
Peppers, green	2	Mulberries, raw	7
Potatoes, boiled	18	Nectarine, raw	10
Potatoes, fried (chips)	34	Oranges	9
oven chips	30	Orange juice	9
roast	26	Peaches	9
Potato crisps	50	canned in syrup	23
Spinach, boiled	1	Pears	11
Sweetcorn, canned	17	Pineapple, canned in juice	12
Sweet potato	22	Plums	8
Tomatoes, fresh	3	Prunes, dried	40
Turnips, cooked	2	Raisins	60
Watercress	1	Raspberries	6
Yam, boiled	30	Rhubarb, cooked, no sugar	1
		Strawberries	6
Fruit		Sultanas	65
Apples	12		
Apricots, canned in syrup	28	**Nuts**	
stewed, no sugar	5	Almonds	4
dried	43	Brazils	4

Food	Carbohydrate
Cashews	27
Coconut, desiccated	6
Hazelnuts	7
Peanuts, roasted, salted	9
Peanut butter	13
Walnuts	3

Cereals

Food	Carbohydrate
Biscuits, chocolate	67
plain, digestive	69
semi-sweet	75
Bread, brown	44
white	49
wholemeal	42
Chelsea bun, (1)	58
Cream crackers	68
Crispbread, rye	71
Flour, white	77
wholemeal	63
Pearl barley	79
Popcorn	66
Rice, raw	86
Spaghetti, raw	74
Tapioca	90

Breakfast cereals

Food	Carbohydrate
Cornflakes	85
Muesli	66
Oats, porridge	66
Weetabix	70

Cakes, pastries

Food	Carbohydrate
Chocolate cake with butter icing	53
Fruit cake, rich	51
Jam tarts	63
Plain cake, Madeira	58

Puddings

Food	Carbohydrate
Apple pie	57
Bread and butter pudding	17
Cheesecake, frozen, fruit topping	33
Custard	17
Ice-cream, dairy	21
Rice pudding	20
Trifle	20

Beverages

Food	Carbohydrate
Chocolate, drinking	77
Cocoa powder	12

NOTE 1. Alcohol. There is some dispute over the effect of alcohol. One theory has it that alcohol reduces the combustion of fat in the body in a similar way to carbohydrate. On the other hand, Banting drank up to six glasses of claret each day and a glass of rum most evenings - and still lost weight. By dilating the blood vessels in the skin, making it work harder, alcohol may step up the metabolism sufficiently to compensate for the added calories taken in the alcohol. There is also experimental evidence that such increased metabolism coupled with increased loss of water from the skin and in urine could result in weight loss.

APPENDIX C
LOW-CARBOHYDRATE MENUS

Notes

The Banting diet is simply a matter of reducing the carbohydrate content of meals. You can eat as much meat, fish, eggs, cheese, butter and cream as you like, only cutting down on foods high in sugars and starches, such as sugar, honey, jam, bread, pasta and potatoes. Thus you do not really need special menus. Those given below are examples where the carbohydrate content has been calculated to give some idea of minimum daily amounts.

Margarine is not recommended for the reasons given in Chapter 6. In the menus which follow, however, margarine may be substituted for butter if you wish. Do not use the low-fat spreads.

Beverages with each meal: water, non-calorie soft drinks, coffee or tea with a little milk or as much cream as desired, sweetened with artificial sweetener if necessary.

DAILY MENUS

Breakfast	Lunch	Dinner
1 cup grapefruit juice	Beef steak with its fat	Poached halibut
herb omelette	½ cup carrots in butter	green salad
2-3 rashers streaky bacon	1 cup green beans	cheese with two
	1 thin slice sponge cake	water biscuits and
1 slice buttered toast		butter.
22 grams	**27 grams**	**11 grams**
	Total carbohydrate for the day: 60 grams	

½ an orange	1 cup consommé	Pork cutlets
scrambled eggs	roast ham	1 cup Brussels
2-3 slices streaky bacon	cucumber and tomato	sprouts with cream
1 slice buttered toast	salad	½ cup carrots
	½ cup fresh fruit, cream	small slice dark fruit cake
20 grams	**20 grams**	**20 grams**
	Total carbohydrate for the day: 60 grams	

Breakfast	**Lunch**	**Dinner**
1 cup tomato juice	Fried plaice	grilled beef steak
scrambled eggs in	medium serving	1 cup spinach with
butter	fried chips	butter or cream
salami	green salad	small portion mashed
1 slice buttered toast	1 fresh peach	potato
		2 soda crackers, butter
		and cheddar cheese
14 grams	**30 grams**	**20 grams**

Total carbohydrate for the day: 64 grams

1 cup orange juice	Corned beef	2 pork chops with fat
scrambled eggs in butter	tomato salad	1 cup mixed vegetables
1 kipper	mayonnaise made	½ cup fresh fruit salad
1 slice buttered toast	with cream	with cream
	cheese and apple	
20 grams	**15 grams**	**25 grams**

Total carbohydrate for the day: 60 grams

½ grapefruit	1 slice melon	Asparagus soup
large portion of white	Beef and vegetable	2 lamb chops, mint sauce
fish, poached in milk,	stew, no potatoes	½ cup carrots
with butter	½ cup french beans	½ cup buttered peas
1 slice buttered toast	Brie or Cheddar cheese	small portion mashed
		potatoes
		peach and cream
17 grams	**15 grams**	**30 grams**

Total carbohydrate for the day: 63 grams

1 cup tomato juice	Oxtail soup	Prawn salad
Mushroom omelette	Tinned salmon or tuna	Roast beef
2-3 rashers streaky	tomato and cucumber	½ cup carrots
bacon	salad	1 cup cabbage
fried kidneys	potato salad	1 roast potato
fried tomatoes	fresh fruit salad with	rhubarb crumble with
1 slice fried bread	cream	cream
17 grams	**15 grams**	**35 grams**

Total carbohydrate for the day: 67 grams

APPENDIX D
MEDICAL REFERENCES

In medical journals, a note of each reference is made with the point it is making in the discussion. As this can tend to distract the reader, these notes have been omitted from this book. However, I believe that the reader should have the opportunity of checking the references. For this reason they are listed below in the order in which they are used.

Large teaching hospitals have medical libraries which are established for the benefit of medical personnel. However, they may be available to members of the general public if permission is sought. Journals are usually stored in alphabetical and date order. There is an *Index Medicus* for each year which indexes all reports, papers, studies, letters, and so on by subject and by author.

Reference formats vary from journal to journal. Those below all follow a standard pattern for ease of use. The format used is: Author, subject, journal, year, volume, (part), first page of article.

Chapter One
Jarrett R J, *Is there an ideal body weight?* Br Med J. 1986; ii: 493.

Lewin R. *Overblown reports distort obesity risks*. Science 1981; 211: 258.

Sours H E, et al. *Sudden death associated with very low calorie weight reduction regimes.* Am J Clin Nutr. 1981; 34: 453.

Liddle R D, et al. *Gallstone formation during weight-reduction dieting.* Arch Intern Med. 1989; 149: 1750.

Moses N, et al. *Fear of obesity among adolescent girls.* Pediatrics. 1989; 83: 393.

Chapter Two
Lee R B. *What hunters do for a living, or how to make out on scarce resources.* In: Lee R B, DeVore I, eds. *Man The Hunter.* Aldine, Chicago. 1968.

– *The !Kung San: men, women and work in a foraging society.* Cambridge University Press, New York. 1979.

Gaulin S J C, Konner M. *On the natural diet of primates, including humans.* In: Wurtman R Y, Wurtman J J, eds. *Nutrition and The Brain.* Vol 1, Raven Press, New York. 1977.

Bryant V M, Williams-Dean G. *The Coprolites of Man.* Scientific American,

January 1975.

Crawford M, Crawford S. *The Food We Eat Today.* Spearman, London, 1972.

Leopold A C. *Toxic Substances in Plants and Food Habits of Early Man.* Science, 1972

Hawkes J G. *The Hunting Hypothesis.* In: Ardrey R, ed. *The Hunting Hypothesis.* Collins, London, 1976.

Yudkin J. *Archaeology and the nutritionist.* In: Ardrey R, ed. *The Hunting Hypothesis.* Collins, London, 1976.

Cleave T L. *The neglect of natural principles in current medical practice.* J RN Med Serv 1956; XLII, No 2: 55.

McGregor-Robertson J. *The Household Physician.* Vol 2. The Gresham Publishing Co. Ltd. London.

Given H D C. *A New Angle on Health.* John Bale, Sons & Danielsson Ltd. 1935.

McClellan W S, Du Bois E F. *Prolonged meat diets with a study of kidney function and ketosis.* J Biol Chem. 1930; 87: 651

Orr J B, Gilks J L. *Studies of Nutrition: The Physique and Health of Two African Tribes.* HMSO, London, 1931.

McCormick J, Elmore-Meegan M. *Maasai Diet.* Lancet 1992; 340: 1042.

Sandler B P. *How to Prevent Heart Attacks.* Lee Foundation for Nutritional Research, Milwarkee, Wisconsin.

Rifkind B M et al. *Effects of short-term sucrose restriction on serum-lipid levels.* Lancet, 24 December 1961.

Yudkin J. *Dietary sucrose and the behaviour of blood platelets.* Proceedings of the Nutrition Society; 29. 1969.

Flint F J. *The factor of infection in heart failure.* Br Med J. 1954; 2: 1018.

How important are respiratory infections as a cause of heart failure? Arteriosclerosis, Sep 7, 1955.

Wilder J. *Nutrition and mental deficiency.* Nervous Child 1944; 3: 174

Makinen K K. *The role of sucrose and other sugars in the development of dental caries: A review.* Int Dent J. 1972; 22 (3): 363.

Cleave T L. *The Saccharine Disease.* Keats Publishing, New Canaan, Conn. 1975.

Ahrens R A. *Sucrose, hypertension and heart disease: A historical perspective.* Am J Clin Nutr. 1974; 27.

Chapter Three

Rose G A, Williams R T. *Metabolic studies on large eaters and small eaters.*

Br J Nutr. 1961; 15: 188

George V, et al. *Further evidence for the presence of 'small eaters' and 'large eaters' among women*. Am J Clin Nutr. 1991; 53: 425.

Jung R T, et al. *Reduced thermogenesis in obesity*. Nature. 1979; 279: 323.

Himms-Hagen J. *Obesity may be due to a malfunctioning of brown fat*. Can Med Assn J. 1979; 121: 1361.

– *Thyroid hormones and thermogenesis*. In *Mammalian Thermogenesis* (Girardier L and Stock N J. Eds) Chapman and Hall, London, 1983.

Rothwell N J, Stock N J. *A role for brown adipose tissue in diet-induced thermogenesis*. Nature. 1979; 281: 31.

Schutz Y, et al. *Diet-induced thermogenesis measured over a whole day in obese and non-obese women*. Am J Clin Nutr. 1984; 40: 542.

Isner J M, et al. *Sudden unexpected deaths in avid dieters using the liquid protein modified fast diet*. Circulation. 1979; 60: 1401.

Chapter Four

Pacy P J, et al. *The energy cost of aerobic exercise in fed and fasted normal subjects*. Am J Clin Nutr. 1985; 42: 764.

Rothwell N J, Stock N J. *Regulation of energy balance*. Ann Rev Nutr. 1981; 1: 235.

Reid R L, van Vugt D A. *Weight-related changes in reproductive function*. Fertil Steril. 1987; 48(6): 905.

Cumming D C, et al. *Exercise and reproductive function in women*. Prog Clin Biol Res. 1983; 117: 113.

– *Defects in pulsatile release in normally menstruating runners*. J Clin Endocrin Metab. 1985; 60(4): 810.

Schwartz B, et al. *Exercise associated amenorrhea: a distinct entity?* Am J Obstet Gynecol. 1981; 141: 662.

Editorial. *Reduced testosterone and prolactin in male distance runners*. J A M A. 1984; 252: 514.

Chalmer J et al. *Anorexia nervosa presenting as morbid exercising*. Lancet. 1985; i: 286.

Coplan N L, Gleim G W, Nicholas J A. *Exercise and sudden cardiac death*. Am Heart J. 1988; 115(1) pt.1: 207.

Fonda J. *Jane Fonda's Workout Book*. Penguin, London, 1984.

Morris J N, et al. *Vigorous exercise in leisure time and the incidence of coronary heart disease*. Lancet. 1973; i: 333.

Wagner W. *Exercise-induced Allergic Syndromes on the Increase*. Cleveland

Clin J Med. 1989; 56: 665.

Selye H. *The Stress of Life.* McGraw-Hill New York 1956.
– *Annual Report on Stress. Montreal.* Acta Inc. 1951; Selye H, Horava A.
1952, 1953; Selye H, Heuser G, 1954; M D Public, New York 1955-56.

Sawrey W L, Weisz J D. *An experimental method of producing gastric ulcers.*
J Comp Physio Psychol. 1956; 49: 269

Solomon G F. *Psychophysiological aspects of rheumatoid arthritis and auto-
immune disease.* In Hill O W (Ed). *Modern Trends in Psychosomatic
Medicine* – 2. Butterworths, London, 1970.

Chapter Five

Mirkin G B, Shore R N. *The Beverly Hills Diet: dangers of the newest weight
loss fad.* J A M A. 1981; 246: 2235.

Van Itallie T B. *The liquid protein mayhem.* J A M A. 1978; 240: 140.

Wadden T A, et al. *The Cambridge Diet: more mayhem?* J A M A 1983; 250:
2283.

Editorial. *Caution: very low calorie diets can be deadly.* Ann Int Med. 1985;
102: 121.

Isner J M, et al. *Sudden unexpected deaths in avid dieters using the liquid
protein modified fast diet.* Circulation. 1979; 60: 1401.

Sours H E, et al. *Sudden death associated with very low calorie weight
reduction regimes.* Am J Clin Nutr. 1981; 34: 453.

Editorial. *In praise of embonpoint.* Lancet. 1987; ii: 491.

Banting W. *Letter on Corpulence to the Public.* 1863.

Densmore H. *How to Reduce Fat.* H Densmore, Los Angeles, 1895.

Stefansson V. *The Fat of The Land.* Macmillan & Co. New York. 1956.

Kekwick A, Pawan G L S. *Calorie intake in relation to body-weight changes
in the obese.* Lancet. 1956; ii: 155.

Hausberger F X, Milstein S W. *Dietary effect on lipogenesis in adipose tissue.*
J Bio Chem. 1955; 214: 483.

Committee on Medical Aspects of Food. *Diet and Cardiovascular Disease.*
DHSS. 1984.

Obesity: a report of the Royal College of Physicians. J R Coll Phys of
London. 1983; 17 (1).

Chapter Six

Strong J P, McGill H C jr. *The natural history of coronary atherosclerosis.*
Am J Pathol. 1962;40:37.

Enos W F, Holmes R H, Beyer J. *Coronary disease among United States soldiers killed in action in Korea. Preliminary report.* JAMA 1953; 152: 1090.

McMichael J M. *Fats and atheroma: an inquest.* Br Med J. 1979; 279: 890.
– *Diet and coronary disease.* Acta Med Scand. 1980; 207(3): 151.

Smith E B, Smith R H. *Early changes in aortic intima.* Atheroscler Rev. 1976; I: 119.

Wass V J, et al. *Does the nephrotic syndrome increase the risk of cardiovascular disease?* Lancet. 1979; ii: 664.

Moore R A. *Variation in serum cholesterol.* Lancet. 1988; ii: 682.

Editorial. *Virus infections and atherosclerosis.* Lancet. 1978; ii: 821.

Houghton J L, von Dohlen T W, Frank MJ. *Myocardial ischaemia without atherosclerosis.* Postgrad Med. 1989; 86 (5): 121.

Woodhill J M et al. *Low fat, low cholesterol diet in secondary prevention of coronary heart disease.* In: D Kritschevky, R Paoletti, W L Holmes Eds *Drugs, lipid metabolism and atherosclerosis.* New York: Plenum Press, 1978: 317.

Diet and Cardiovascular Disease. Committee on Medical Aspects of Food. DHSS. 1984.

Kannel WB, Gordon T. *The Framingham Diet Study: diet and the regulations of serum cholesterol (Sect 24).* Washington DC, Dept of Health, Education and Welfare, 1970.

Kannel W B, Castelli.W P. *Is serum cholesterol an anachronism?* Lancet. 1979; 2: 950.

Nichols A B, et al. *Daily nutritional intake and serum lipid levels: The Tecumseh Study.* Am J Clin Nutr. 1976; 29: 1384.

Multiple Risk Factor Intervention Trial. J A M A. 1982; 248: 1465.

World Health Organisation. European Collaborative Group. *Multi-factorial trial in the prevention of coronary heart disease: 3. Incidence and mortality results.* Eur Heart J. 1983; 4: 141

Salonen J T, et al. *Changes in morbidity and mortality during comprehensive community programme to control cardiovascular diseases during 1972-1977 in North Karelia.* Br Med J. 1979; iv: 1178.

Puska P. *The North Karelia Project: a community based programme for the prevention of heart and vascular disease.* Duodecim (Helsinki). 1985; 101(23): 2281.

Lipid Research Clinic Programme. *LRC-CPPT results. Reduction in incidence of coronary heart disease.* J A M A. 1984; 251: 351.

Ravnskov V. *Cholesterol lowering trials in coronary heart disease: frequency of citation and outcome.* Br Med J. 1992; 305: 15.

Gortner W A. *Nutrition in the United States, 1900 to 1974.* Cancer Res. 1975; 35: 3246.

Barker D J P, Osmond C. *Diet and coronary heart disease in England and Wales during and after the second world war.* J Epidemiol Com Hlth. 1986; 40: 37

McKeigne P M, Miller G P, Marmot M G. *Coronary heart disease in South Asians overseas: A review.* J Clin Epidemiol. 1989; 42(7): 597.

Marmot M G. *Interpretation of Trends in Coronary Heart Disease Mortality.* Acta Med Scand. 1985 (Suppl); 701: 58.

Beaglehole et al. *Cholesterol and mortality in New Zealand Maoris.* Br Med J. 1980; 1: 285.

Ahrens E H. *Dietary fats and coronary heart disease: unfinished business.* Lancet. 1979; ii: 1345.

Dedichen J. T Norske Laegeforen. 1976; 16: 915.

Pearce M L, Dayton S. *Incidence of cancer in men on a diet high in polyunsaturated fat.* Lancet. 1971; i: 464.

Hofmann A F, Northfield T C, Thistle J L. *Can a cholesterol-lowering diet cause gallstones?* New Eng J Med. 1973; 288 (1): 46.

Willett W C, et al. *Intake of trans fatty acids and risk of coronary heart disease among women.* Lancet 1993; 341: 581.

Carroll K K. *Dietary fats and cancer.* Am J Clin Nutr 1991; 53: 1064S.

France T, Brown P. *Test-tube cancers raise doubts over fats.* New Scientist, December 7, 1991, p 12.

Kearney R. *Promotion and prevention of tumour growth – effects of endotoxin, inflammation and dietary lipids.* Int Clin Nutr Rev 1987; 7: 157.

Burkitt D P et al. *Some geographical variations in disease patterns in East and Central Africa.* E Afr Med J. 1963; 40: 1.

Trowell H C. *Fibre and irritable bowels.* Br Med J. 1974; 3: 44.

– *Dietary fibre, ischaemic heart disease and diabetes mellitus.* Proc Nutr Soc. 1973; 32: 151.

Swain F, et al. *Comparison of the effects of oat bran and low-fiber wheat on serum lipoprotein levels and blood pressure.* New Eng J Med. 1990; 322(3): 147.

Connor W E. *Dietary fiber – nostrum or critical nutrient?* New Eng J Med. 1990; 322 (3): 193.

Marshall E. *Diet Advice, with a Grain of Salt and a Large Helping of Pepper.*

Science. 1986; 231: 537.

Lichtenstein M J, et al. *Heart rate, employment status and prevalent ischaemic heart disease confound relationship between cereal fibre intake and blood pressure.* J of Epid and Community Health. 1986; 40(4): 330.

Norman D, et al. *The impact of dietary fat and fibre on intestinal carcinogenesis.* Prev Med. 1987; (4): 554.

MacDonald I. *Nonsense and non-science in nutrition.* Proc Nutr Soc. 1983; 42: 513

Anon. Br Med J. 1986; 292: 494.

Kelsay J L. *A review of research on effect of fibre intake on man.* Am J of Clin Nutr. 1978; (31): 142.

Kaneko K et al. *Effect of fibre on protein, fat and calcium digestibilities and fecal cholesterol excretion.* J Nutr Sci Vitaminol (Tokyo). 1986; 32(3): 317.

Kritchevsky D. *Fibre and cancer.* in (Vahouny G V and Kritchevsky D Eds.) *Dietary Fibre: Basic and Clinical Aspects.* Plenum, NY. 1986. p427.
– *Dietary studies of cancer of the large bowel in the animal model.* Ibid p469.

Gerutti G, et al. *Phytic acid in bran and in 'natural' foods.* Bolletino Chimico Farmaceutico, Milan.

Stevens J, et al. *Effect of psyllium gum and wheat bran on spontaneous energy intake.* Am J Clin Nutr. 1987; 46: 812.

Editorial. *The Bran Wagon.* Lancet. 1987; i: 782.

Suri Y P. *The Bran Wagon.* Lancet. 1987; ii: 42.

Bindra G S, Gibson R S. *Iron status of predominantly lacto-ovo-vegetarian East Indian immigrants to Canada: a model approach.* Am J Clin Nutr. 1986; 44: 643.

Turnlund J R, et al. *A stable isotope study of zinc absorption in young men: effects of phytate and alpha-cellulose.* Am J Clin Nutr. 1984; 40: 1071.

Sandstrom B, et al. *The effects of vegetables and beet fibre on the absorption of zinc in humans from composite meals.* Br J Nutr. 1987; 58 (1): 49.

Hallberg L, et al. *Phytates and the inhibitory effect of bran on iron absorption in man.* Am J Clin Nutr. 1987; 45(5): 988.

Balasubraminian R, et al. *Effect of wheat bran on bowel function and fecal calcium in older adults.* J Am Coll Nutr. 1987; 6(3): 199.

Hallfisch J, et al. *Mineral balances of men and women consuming high fibre diets with complex or simple carbohydrate.* J Nutr. 1987; 117(2): 403.

Fractured neck of femur: prevention and management. A report of the Royal College of Physicians, London. 1989.

Editorial: *Why so many fractured hips?* Lancet. 1989; i: 57.

Fehily A M,. *Dietary determinants of bone mass and fracture risk: a review.* J Hum Nutr and Diet. 1989; 2: 299.

Wargovich M J, Baer A R. *Basic and Clinical Investigations of Dietary Calcium in the Prevention of Colorectal Cancer.* Prev Med. 1989; 18: 672.

BBC. Horizon: *The Poison That Waits.* BBC2 broadcast 16 Jan 1989.

Bishop N, McGraw M, Ward N. *Aluminium in infant formulas.* Lancet. 1989; i: 490.

Golden B E, Golden M H N. *Plasma zinc, rate of weight gain and the energy cost of tissue deposition in children recovering from malnutrition on cows' milk or a soya protein based diet.* Am J Clin Nutr. 1981; 34: 892.

Prasad A. *The role of zinc in gastrointestinal and liver disease.* Clin Gastroenterol. 1983; 12: 713.

Aggett P, Davies N. *Some nutritional aspects of trace elements.* J Inter Metab Dis. 1983; 6(2): 22.

Hambidge M. *The role of zinc and other trace metals in paediatric nutrition and health.* Paediat Clin N Am. 1977; 24: 95.

Bryce-Smith D, Simpson R. *Anorexia, depression and zinc deficiency.* Lancet. 1984; ii: 1162.

Fonesca V, Harvard C. *Electrolyte disturbances and cardiac failure with hypomagnesaemia in anorexia nervosa.* Br Med J. 1985; 291: 1680

Meadows N, et al. *Zinc and small babies.* Lancet. 1981; ii: 1135.

Bryce-Smith D. *Environmental chemical influences on behaviour and mentation.* John Jeyes lecture. Chem Soc Rev. 1986; 15: 93.

McMichael A, et al. *A prospective study of serial maternal zinc levels and pregnancy outcome.* Early Human Development. 1982 (Elsevier); 7: 59.

Addy D. *Happiness is: iron.* Br Med J. 1986; 292: 969

Luk'ianova E M. *Diagnosis of vitamin D deficiency rickets.* Pediatriia. 1988;(3):15.

Adelman R. *Nutritional rickets.* Am J Dis Child. 1988; 142(4): 414.

Clements M R. *The problem of rickets in UK Asians.* J Hum Nutr Diet, 1989; 2: 105.

Hughes R E. *A new look at dietary fibre.* Hum Nutr Clin Nutr. 1986; 40c: 81.

Hughes R E, Johns E. *Apparent relation between dietary fibre and reproductive function in the female.* Ann Hum Biol. 1985; 12: 325.

Lloyd T, et al. *Inter-relationships of diet, athletic activity, menstrual status and bone density in collegiate women.* Am J Clin Nutr. 1987; 46: 681.

Southgate D A T. *Minerals, trace elements and potential hazards.* Am J Clin

Nutr. 1987; 45: 1256.

Yusuf S, Furberg C D. *Single factor trials: control through lifestyle changes.* In A G Olsson, ed. *Atherosclerosis.* Edinburgh: Churchill-Livingstone, 1987: 389.

Lipid Research Clinics *Coronary Primary Prevention Trial: I. Reduction in incidence of coronary heart disease. II. The relationship of reduction in incidence of coronary heart disease to cholesterol lowering.* J A M A. 1984; 251: 351.

Committee of Principle Investigators: *World Health Organization cooperative trial on primary prevention of ischaemic heart disease using clofibrate to lower serum cholesterol: the final mortality follow up.* Lancet. 1984; ii: 379.

Frick M F, et al. *Helsinki Heart Study: primary prevention trial with gemfibrozil in middle aged men with dyslipidemia.* New Eng J Med. 1987; 317: 1237.

Coronary Drug Project Research Group: *Gall bladder disease as a side effect of drugs influencing lipid metabolism.* New Eng J Med. 1977; 296: 1185.

Dukes M N G. *Drugs affecting lipid metabolism.* in: M N G Dukes ed. *Meyler's Side Effects of Drugs,* Ninth Edition. Excerpta Medica, Amsterdam, 1980.

Yusuf S, Cutler J. *Single factor trials: drug studies.* in A G Olsson, ed. *Atherosclerosis.* Edinburgh: Churchill-Livingstone, 1987: 389.

Davey Smith G, Song F, Sheldon T A. *Cholesterol lowering and mortality: the importance of considering initial level of risk.* Br Med J. 1993; 306: 1367.

McMichael A J, et al. *Dietary and endogenous cholesterol and human cancer.* Epidemiol Rev. 1984; 6: 192.

Cambien F, et al. *Total serum cholesterol and cancer mortality in a middle aged male population.* Am J Epid. 1980; 112: 388.

Garcia-Palmieri M R, et al. *An apparent inverse relationship between serum cholesterol and cancer mortality in Puerto Rico.* Am J Epid. 1981; 114: 29.

Kozarevic D, et al. *Serum cholesterol and mortality: the Yugoslavian cardiovascular diseases study.* Am J Epid. 1981; 114: 21.

Hiatt R A, Fireman B H. *Serum cholesterol and the incidence of cancer in a large cohort.* J Chronic Dis. 1986; 39: 861.

Schatzkin A, et al. *Serum cholesterol and cancer in the NHANES I epidemiologic follow up study.* Lancet. 1987; ii: 298.

Kagan A, et al. *Serum cholesterol and mortality in a Japanese-American population: the Honolulu heart program.* Am J Epid. 1981; 114: 11.

Isles C G, et al. *Plasma cholesterol, coronary heart disease and cancer in the Renfrew and Paisley survey.* Br Med J. 1989; 298: 920.

Winawer S J, et al. *Declining Serum Cholesterol Levels Prior to Diagnosis of Colon Cancer.* JAMA. 1990; 263 (15): 2083.

Takashi Shimamoto, et al. *Trends for Coronary Heart Disease and Stroke and Their Risk Factors in Japan.* Circulation. 1989; 3: 503.

Cholesterol in the prediction of atherosclerotic disease: new perspectives based on the Framingham Study. Ann Int Med. 1979; 90: 85.

Corrigan FM et al. *Dietary supplementation with zinc sulphate, sodium selenite and fatty acids in early dementia of Altzheimer's Type II: Effects on lipids.* J Nutr Med 1991; 2: 265.

Hulley S et al. *Editorial on Conference on low blood cholesterol.* Circulation 1992; 86 (3): 1026.

Report on the US National Heart, Lung and Blood Institute Conference on low blood cholesterol: Mortality associations. Circulation 1992; 86 (3): 1046.

Oliver M F. *Reducing Cholesterol Does Not Reduce Mortality.* JACC. 1988; 12 (3): 814.

McCormick J, Skrabanek P. *Coronary heart disease is not preventable by population interventions.* Lancet. 1988; ii: 839.

Bachorik P S, Cloey T A, Finney C A, Lowry D R, Becker D M. *Lipoprotein-cholesterol analysis during screening: accuracy and reliability.* Ann Intern Med. 1991; 114: 741.

Myers G L et al. *College of American Pathologists – Centres for Disease Control collaborative study for evaluating reference materials for total serum cholesterol measurement.* Arch Pathol Lab Med. 1990; 114: 1199.

Cochrane A L, Holland W W. *Validation of screening procedures.* Brit Med Bull. 1971; 27: 3.

Sharp I, Rayner M. *Cholesterol testing with desk-top machines.* Lancet. 1990; i: 55.

Registrar General's Mortality (Cause) Statistics 1971, 1991.

Chapter Eight

Heaton K W. *Breakfast – do we need it? Report of meeting of Forum on Food and Health, 16 June 1989.* J Royal Soc Med. 1989; 82: 770.

Orent-Keiles E, Hallman L F. *The Breakfast Meal in Relation to Blood Sugar Values.* US Department of Agriculture Circular No 827 (1949).

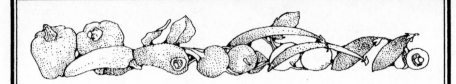

THE CALORIE FALLACY RECIPES

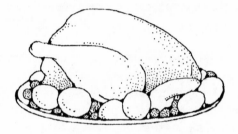

High-calorie, low-carbohydrate recipes for weight loss

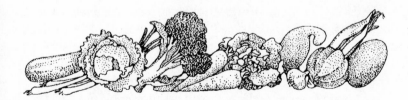

LOW-CARBOHYDRATE RECIPES

Introduction
People become overweight, not because they eat too much but because they eat too much of the wrong food. Both Man's history and clinical medical trials have proved that *only* carbohydrates are fattening. Most slimming diets reduce fat intake or cut out fats altogether. Eating fat, however, has been shown time and time again to speed up weight loss – the fact is that fat is slimming.

To lose weight it is only necessary to reduce your intake of carbohydrates to about 60 grams a day. The recipes here may contain far more calories than you are used to finding in a slimming diet, but they are all low in carbohydrates.

Food types
The science of nutrition is absorbing if you have the time to study it; but most of us do not. You do not need to be a qualified nutritionist to eat healthily. It is useful, however, to know something about what your body needs.

Foods are split into three main types: proteins, fats and carbohydrates. The body also needs very small amounts of a variety of other nutrients: minerals, vitamins and trace elements.

Protein is the body's building material. It is used to make new tissue as we grow and to repair tissue as we continue through life. Therefore protein is an essential part of any diet. The body needs an adequate supply of complete proteins throughout the day and every day. The principal sources of complete proteins are: animal foods such as meat, fish, eggs, milk and cheese, and soya bean. Vegetables, notably cereals, pulses (peas, beans and lentils) and nuts also supply proteins. Generally these are incomplete: vegetables of the various groups have to eaten together in the correct proportion to provide the body with complete proteins.

Fats are used to provide energy and heat. Thus they are of particular importance during the winter. However, they are also precursors for a number of other body functions and, as such, a certain amount of fat in the diet is essential. The principal sources of fat are: butter and margarine, cooking fats, animal fat, cream, cheese, oily fish and fish liver oils, nuts, and olive oil.

Carbohydrates split into two main groups: starches and sugars. Both groups are turned to sugar in the body and used to supply energy. They have no structural uses. The main sources of the starches are: all cereals such as wheat, barley, rice and oats; flour and bread, cakes, biscuits; vegetables such as potatoes and parsnips. Sugars are found in sugar, honey, jam, marmalade, sweets, sweet fruit and some root vegetables, e.g., beetroot and carrot.

Vitamins, minerals and trace elements are also required in small amounts. Provided that a western-style diet – high in animal products, green vegetables both cooked and uncooked, and fruit – is eaten, there is little risk of a deficiency occurring.

Recipes

The breakfast recipes which follow are designed to fill and satisfy, to get you off to a good start. This is all important if you are to function at your best.

The ideas for lunches are aimed at the working man or woman who needs to carry a packed lunch to eat at the workplace.

As you only need to reduce your intake of carbohydrates to lose weight, dinners can probably consist of the foods you eat now with, say, more meat and less potato. Therefore the dinner recipes are gourmet ones for dinner parties or special occasions.

Breakfast Recipes

As it comes at the end of a ten or eleven hour fast, breakfast is the most important meal of the day. Ignore it and the body may have to wait a further 4 or 5 hours. In this situation, the body cannot function properly. Not only will you be less energetic and mentally alert, such a long period without nourishment can harm the body's energy regulating mechanisms. Any breakfast is better than none but for peak efficiency you need to start the day with a good supply of nutrients.

Cold breakfasts, based on cold meats, hard-boiled eggs and cheeses, can be prepared the day before they are needed. If you enjoy a cooked breakfast, however, it is worth taking the little extra time it takes to prepare and cook one. An easy and quick breakfast is the traditional bacon and eggs. To fry these takes about 10 minutes, only makes one pan dirty and contains no carbohydrate.

Always use lard, beef dripping or other animal fat for frying or grilling. When heated, vegetable oils which are high in polyunsaturated fats oxidise readily, can cause free radicals to form and are potent promoters of cancers. It is unwise to use vegetable-based 'cooking' oils, such as sunflower oil, for cooking at high temperature: frying, grilling or roasting. If you must use oil, olive oil is safer.

Most of the recipes below do not include bread or toast. If you include bread, reckon its carbohydrate content at 12 grams per slice.

The figures given for carbohydrate content are reckoned per person.

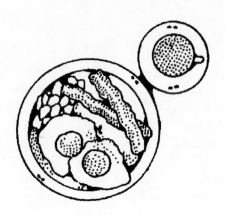

Mixed Grill

4 slices lamb's liver	salt and black pepper
4 lamb's kidneys	4 tomatoes, halved
40 g (1½ ozs) lard	8 large mushrooms

Skin and core the kidneys and halve them lengthwise.

Line a grill pan with foil and melt the lard and spread in it. Put the liver in the middle of the pan surrounded with the kidneys. Brush with lard.

Grill under a medium heat until the liver and kidneys change colour (approx 3 mins), and turn them over. Sprinkle with salt and pepper to taste.

Arrange the tomatoes and mushrooms around the kidneys, with the cut sides of tomatoes and caps of mushrooms uppermost. Sprinkle them with salt and pepper and brush with fat.

Grill for a further 5 minutes and serve hot.

Serves 4.   **Carbohydrate: 3 grams.**

Kidneys à l'orange

4 sheep's kidneys
25 g (1 oz) butter
1 shallot
2 mushrooms
salt and pepper
1 tsp flour

½ pint stock
orange peel, grated
4 slices of toast
butter
orange peel, grated

Cut the kidneys in half, lengthwise, skin them and remove the white parts (if using ox kidneys, cut into pieces). Melt the butter in a deep frying pan or a saucepan, put in the kidneys and fry brown. Chop the shallot and mushrooms small and add to the kidneys, season with salt and pepper. When these have fried brown, stir in the flour and brown this. Pour in the stock and simmer for about 20 minutes, with the lid off to reduce the stock. Flavour with grated orange peel and serve hot on a slice of buttered toast.
Serves 4.   **Carbohydrate: 13 grams.**

Poached Eggs on Toast

300 ml (½ pint) of water
pinch of salt
4 eggs

2 slices white bread
butter
1 tsp yeast extract

Put the water and salt in an egg poacher and bring to the boil. Break the eggs into the poacher and simmer for three minutes until the eggs are set. Toast the bread lightly on both sides, then spread with butter and yeast extract. Remove the eggs and place on top of the toast.
Serves 2.   **Carbohydrate: 12 grams.**

Scrambled Eggs

4 eggs
4 tbsp single cream
salt
white pepper

butter
2 slices white bread
2 tsp chopped chives

2 tsp chopped parsley. Break the eggs into a bowl, add the cream and salt and pepper to taste. Whisk with a fork until mixed.

Melt some butter in a small saucepan. Add the egg mixture and cook gently, stirring constantly, until the eggs begin to set, but are not fully set. Use a low light or lift the pan occasionally.

At the same time, toast the bread lightly and spread with butter. While the eggs are setting but still creamy, stir in the chives and parsley. Pile onto the toast and serve immediately.

Serves 2.   **Carbohydrate: 13 grams.**

Breakfast Omelettes

These are basic omelettes with a variety of toppings. You could use the toppings listed below one at a time or combine them for variety.

Basic ingredients	Toppings	
2 eggs per person	streaky bacon	cooked ham
1 tbsp milk or cream	mushrooms	Cheddar cheese
salt and black pepper	anchovies	cottage cheese
lard or butter	tomatoes	herbs

Break the eggs into a small bowl, add the cream or milk and salt and pepper to taste, and beat until frothy.

Melt the lard or butter into a frying pan and pour in the egg mixture. Cook over a moderate heat until it becomes firm.

When the omelette starts to set, spread the topping onto it and continue cooking until the omelette is set. Fold in half and serve.

Toppings. The cooked ham should be cut small before adding the Cheddar cheese grated before adding. If cottage cheese is used, some may be mixed with the omelette mixture in place of the milk. The bacon should be cut into small pieces and fried first, the omelette mixture being poured over it.

Serves 1.   **Carbohydrate: negligible.**

Baked Ham, Egg and Tomato

4 tomatoes large enough to hold an egg.	4 eggs
100 g (4 oz) cooked ham	salt and pepper
1 tsp chopped parsley	

Cut the tops off the tomatoes and scoop out the seeds and pulp. Remove the seeds from the pulp with a sieve. Mix the ham, parsley and pulp in a bowl with added salt and pepper to taste.

Divide the mixture and put into the tomatoes, pressing it well down. With the tomatoes in a baking dish, break an egg into each and sprinkle with salt and pepper to taste.

Bake in a preheated oven at moderate heat (190°C/375°F/Gas Mark 5) until the eggs are set (about 15 minutes). Serve immediately.

Serves 4.   **Carbohydrate: 3 grams.**

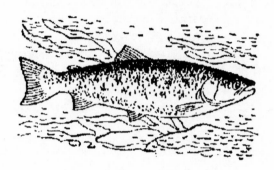

Poached Haddock with Egg

1 lb (450 g) smoked haddock fillets   black pepper
1 pint (600 ml) water   1 oz (25 g) butter
4 eggs

In a frying pan, cover the fish with water. Bring slowly to the boil and simmer until the fish is tender but not breaking up (about 10-15 minutes). Transfer to warm plates and keep hot.

Break an egg into a cup.

Using the cooking water, stir it briskly to create a whirlpool and carefully slide the egg into the water. Simmer until the egg is set (about 3 minutes) Repeat for the other eggs..

Cut the fish into 4 portions, sprinkle with pepper to taste and melt the butter on to it. Place one egg on each piece and serve immediately.

Serves 4.   **Carbohydrate: negligible.**

Kippers and Scrambled Eggs

2 kipper fillets   salt and pepper
4 eggs   butter
milk or cream

Prepare the kippers: wash them well, cut off the head and just cover with boiling water. Cook gently for 2-3 minutes, drain and serve with a knob of butter.

Alternatively, brush with butter and grill for 5-6 minutes.

The kippers may also be fried in lard for 5-7 minutes.

Mix the eggs with a little milk or cream, and salt and pepper to taste. Heat some butter in a saucepan. In it cook the egg mixture, stirring, until it is just set. This should be done while the kippers are cooking. Serve together immediately.

Serves 2   **Carbohydrate: 0**

Fish Omelette

This dish is a useful way of using up leftovers of a fish dish from the previous day. Any white fish may be used.

Remains of cold boiled white fish   1 tbsp milk or cream
4 eggs   40 g (1½ oz) butter
a little white sauce   salt and cayenne pepper

Remove any skin and bones from the fish and break it into small flakes. Melt a little butter in a frying pan, add the fish, seasonings and enough white sauce to moisten the fish. Keep it hot.

Slightly beat the eggs in a basin, add the milk and season to taste. Melt a full 30 grams (ounce) of butter in an omelette pan or small frying pan, pour in the eggs and stir over a high heat until the mixture begins to set. Then release from the bottom of the pan, put the prepared fish in the middle, fold the omelette over, allow it to colour, then serve immediately.

Serves 2.   **Carbohydrate: negligible.**

Lunch Recipes

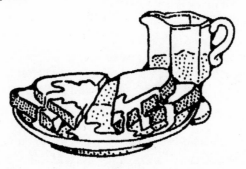

If lunches are eaten at home, their preparation and serving should present few problems. The dinner recipes which follow are equally applicable as lunches. These days, however, many people are away from home at lunchtime. This can make meal preparation more difficult. If you take your lunch in a restaurant or works' canteen, it is safest to choose meat, fish or cheese salads. Eat the lettuce, tomatoes, coleslaw et cetera, but go easy on the potato salad. You could also have a hot meal of, say, roast beef, green vegetables and a little mashed potato, but decline the Yorkshire pudding and go easy on the puddings: finish with cheese rather than a sweet. If you eat in a pub, and normally have a drink, bear in mind the carbohydrate content of the alcohol. Have, say, a whisky highball with soda, a vodka martini or a glass of dry wine – and restrict yourself to just the one.

If you normally take a packed lunch of sandwiches, however, it is not so easy. The ideas for lunches below, therefore, concentrate on meals to be eaten in an office or building site.

Sandwiches

Sandwiches should be used as sparingly as possible, and then be restricted to two slices of bread (carbohydrate content: 24 grams) at any one meal, spread liberally with butter. The secret is to ensure that what fills the sandwich is enough to fill you. The bread may be fresh or toasted.

Fillings.

Cold beef, cut thickly with mustard and a slice of cheese
Minced mutton and mint sauce
Fried bacon and chopped pickled onions

Cheddar cheese and sliced onions
Cooked white fish with pickled walnuts
Grilled cheese on bacon.
Cheese, ham and chicken slices.
2 egg omelette with diced kidney and basil.
Scrambled egg with anchovy paste and chopped watercress
Smoked cods' roes with tomato, lettuce and lemon juice
White fish with tomato sauce

Packed lunches other than sandwiches can be taken to work in covered plastic boxes and eaten either with the fingers or a knife and fork. These can reduce the necessity for bread and, thus, the carbohydrate content.

Finger Salads
If the constituents of a salad are dry, they may be eaten with the fingers.
4 oz (100 g) full-fat cheese, (Cheddar, Brie, Gouda, Edam, etc.) or
4 oz (100 g) cooked sliced ham rolled around a soft cheese such as Philadelphia or
chicken legs or
hard-boiled eggs or
any mixture of the above
with a salad composed of, say, a stick of celery, 1 tomato, ½ green pepper and 1 raw carrot.
Carbohydrate content: approx 10 grams.

A similar meal, replacing the cheese with an individual pork pie, or egg and bacon flan, would have a carbohydrate content of about 20 grams.

Knife and Fork Meals
Salads to be eaten with a knife and fork can be more adventurous. The basis may be any cold meat; lamb cutlets, boiled bacon, chicken legs; fish such as sardines, salmon or tuna; hard-boiled eggs and/or cheese, together with a dressed salad (see Salads and Dressings below). Carbohydrate content will be approximately 13 grams.

Dinner Recipes

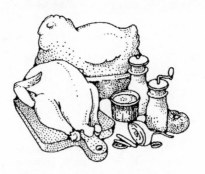

Dinner menus can probably be similar to those you enjoy now. All you may need to do is exclude or reduce the amount of potatoes, pasta, pastry and bread (it is better to cut out pasta, and bread), and compensate by eating more meat, fish, eggs and cheese. These ingredients, with about a cupful in total of root vegetables: onions and carrots, and unlimited green vegetables, is a rough guide. For that reason, the recipes given below are for more special meals when entertaining.

Starters

Tomato Sorbet

340 ml (12 fl oz) tomato juice   2 tsp lemon juice
1 tsp Worcestershire sauce   1 tbsp fresh basil leaves

In a bowl, mix all the ingredients, and salt and pepper to taste. Freeze the mixture in an ice-cube tray until it is firm but not hard.
Serves 2.   **Carbohydrate: 6 grams.**

Chopped Liver with Peanut and Onion

220 g (8 oz) chicken livers, chopped   1 medium onion,
2 tbsp peanut oil   1 hard boiled egg, chopped

In a frying pan, heat the peanut oil until it is hot but not smoking and sauté the chicken livers and onion over a moderately high heat until the liver is cooked right through. Transfer the mixture to a food processor, add the egg and salt and pepper to taste, and blend until the mixture is smooth. Serve on a bed of lettuce with buttered starch-reduced bread or Energen rolls.
Serves 4.   **Carbohydrate: 3 grams.**

Asparagus and Peppers in Mustard Sauce

450 g (1 lb) asparagus, trimmed
1 tbsp tarragon vinegar
1 tbsp Dijon mustard
a dash of Tabasco, to taste
¼ tsp Worcestershire sauce

¼ tsp dried thyme, crumbled
¼ tsp dried tarragon, crumbled
½ cup extra-virgin olive oil
2 sweet red peppers.

Cook the asparagus in boiling salted water until tender (6-8 minutes), and refresh it under cold water.

Dressing. In a bowl, whisk together the vinegar, mustard, Tabasco, Worcestershire sauce, thyme, tarragon and add salt and black pepper to taste. Add the oil in a stream, whisking, and whisk until it is emulsified.

Using a long-handled fork, char the peppers under the grill, turning them every few minutes, until the skin is blistered (15-20 minutes). Transfer to a bowl and allow to steam until cool enough to handle. Keeping them whole, cut off the tops and discard the seeds and ribs.

Divide the asparagus between two plates, arrange the red pepper on it and drizzle the dressing over it.

Serves 2.　　　　　　　　　　　　　　**Carbohydrate: 8 grams.**

Soups

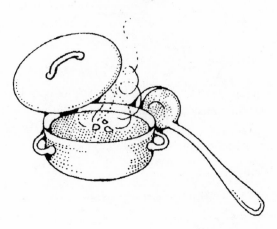

These days, tinned soups are easy to use and the labels give their carbohydrate content. To determine individual carbohydrate content, divide that figure by the number of people having the soup.

However, for something a little different, or if you prefer to make your own, try the ones below.

Cold Prawn Soup

2 pints milk
2 tsp dried English mustard
1 tsp salt
1 tsp sugar
250 g (½ lb) prawns, cooked, cooled and chopped, reserving 2-3

whole prawns halved lengthwise for garnish
1 cucumber, peeled, seeded and chopped fine, reserving a 4-6 slices for garnish if required
2 tbsp minced fresh chives

In a large bowl, whisk together the milk, mustard, salt and sugar. Add the prawns, chopped cucumber and chives and stir until well mixed. Chill the soup, covered for 3 hours in the refrigerator. Garnish each serving with half a prawn and a slice of cucumber

Serves 4-6.   **Carbohydrate: 4 grams.**

Cool Cucumber and Avocado Soup

225 ml (8 fl oz) milk

2 cucumbers, peeled, seeded and chopped

1 avocado, peeled and pitted

2 tbsp chicken stock

2 tbsp lemon juice

¼ tsp ground cumin

In a large measuring jug, mix the milk and sufficient ice cubes to measure 350 ml (12 fl oz) in total. In a blender, blend the milk mixture, half the cucumber, avocado, stock, lemon juice and cumin until the mixture is smooth. Divide between two soup dishes and mix in the remaining cucumber.

Serves 2.   **Carbohydrate: 14 grams.**

Chicken and Egg Soup

1 ltr (2 pints) chicken stock

100-200 g (4-8 oz) ground almonds

6 chicken breasts, chopped finely

6 eggs

salt and pepper

6 bread rolls

Bring the stock to the boil. Add the almonds and chicken and simmer for 15 minutes.

At the same time, cut a hole in the bread rolls and scoop out most of the centre. Crisp the shells in the oven. Strain the soup and fill the rolls with the chopped chicken. Keep warm

Put the remainder of the chicken in the soup and purée in a blender. Reheat, adding salt and pepper to taste.

Poach the eggs.

Place a filled roll with an egg on top in each of six soup bowls, pour the hot soup over and serve.

Serves 6.   **Carbohydrate: 13 grams**

This soup may be used as a main course.

Fish dishes

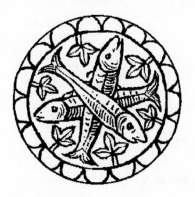

Scallops in Saffron

$\frac{1}{8}$ tsp crumbled saffron threads
2 shallots, minced
15 g (½ oz) butter
1 tbsp white wine vinegar
1 tbsp dry vermouth
2 tbsp double cream
50 g (2 oz) cream cheese

8 large scallops
plain flour for dredging the scallops
50 g (2 oz) lard
½ sweet red pepper cut into julienne
  strips
8 spinach leaves, washed and dried
2 tbsp grated Parmesan

In a small saucepan cook the saffron and the shallot in the butter over a low heat for 2 minutes, or until the saffron begins to dissolve, stirring continuously. Add the vinegar and the vermouth until the mixture is reduced to about 1 tablespoon. Add the cream, bring to the boil and whisk in the cheese. Boil until it is thickened slightly (about 2 minutes), add salt and white pepper to taste. Keep the sauce warm, covered.

Dredge the scallops in the flour, shaking off the excess. In a frying pan, heat the lard over a moderate heat, until it is hot but not smoking. In it sauté the scallops for 1-1½ minutes each side, or until they are browned slightly. Add the pepper and spinach and sauté the mixture, stirring, for 3 minutes, or until the scallops are cooked right through. Pour the sauce into a gratin dish and spoon the scallops and vegetables onto the sauce. Sprinkle the mixture with Parmesan and grill under a pre-heated grill, about 100 mm (4 inches) from the heat until the gratin is just golden on top (about 2 minutes).

Serves 2.   **Carbohydrate: 6 grams.**

Trout with Pine Nuts

4 300 g (10 oz) trout fillets

white pepper to taste

flour for dredging the fillets

25 g (1 oz) clarified butter

100 g (4 oz) butter, melted

25 g (1 oz) pine nuts, toasted lightly

2 tbsp dry white wine

1 tbsp minced chives

1 tbsp minced fresh parsley

pinch of dried thyme

2 tsp lemon juice

Season the fillets with the pepper and salt and dredge them in the flour, shaking off any excess. In a large frying pan, heat the clarified butter over a moderately high heat until it is hot but not smoking. and sauté the fillets in it skin side up for 2 minutes. Turn the fillets and sauté for 2 more minutes. Transfer them to dinner plates.

To the frying pan add the melted butter, and the pine nuts and cook over a moderate heat, swirling it until the butter begins to brown. Remove the pan from the heat, stir in the wine, chives, parsley, thyme and lemon juice and salt to taste. Spoon over the fillets and serve.

Serves 4.   **Carbohydrate: 2 grams.**

Cold Glazed Salmon

½ cup dry white wine

4 basil leaves

1 tarragon sprig plus extra for garnish

1 sprig of rosemary

2 sprigs of celery leaves

2 shallots, minced

1 slice of lemon

1½ kg (3 lb) salmon

1 l (1¾ pints) fish aspic (recipe below)

thin slices of turnip cut in flower shapes for garnish (keep in cold water to prevent discolouring)

1 hard boiled egg yolk mashed with 1 tsp butter for garnish.

In a small saucepan, mix the wine, basil, tarragon, rosemary and celery sprigs, shallots and lemon. Simmer for 15 minutes or until the mixture is reduced to about 1 tablespoon.

Lie the salmon on a sheet of foil which is twice as long as the fish on a baking tray. Raise the edges of the foil and pour the wine mixture over the fish. Season with salt. Fold the foil to enclose the salmon and crimp the edges tightly to secure them.

Bake in the middle of a preheated oven at 190°C/375°F/Gas Mark 5 for 30 minutes or until the flesh just flakes. Transfer to a work surface and remove the foil carefully. Remove the skin from the fish. Drain the liquid from the foil and, using the foil as a guide, turn the fish over onto a plate and skin the other side. Chill the salmon, covered, for at least 4 hours or overnight. Spoon a thin coat of cool but liquid fish aspic over the salmon and arrange the tarragon sprigs and turnip flowers decoratively on the salmon. Spoon a thin coat of cool but liquid fish aspic over the decorations, place a spot of the egg yolk mixture on the centres of the flowers. Chill the salmon for at least 2 hours and serve it with the chilled aspic chopped.

Fish aspic:

450 g (1 lb) white fish trimmings and bones	2 sprigs of tarragon
½ cup dry white wine	2 sprigs of parsley
1 tbsp fresh lemon juice	1 bay leaf
1 medium onion, sliced	75 g (3 oz) unflavoured gelatine
	white and shell of the egg.

In a saucepan, mix the white fish trimmings and bones, wine, lemon juice, onions, tarragon, parsley, tarragon and bay, bring to the boil, stirring frequently to prevent scorching, and boil until it is reduced by half. Add 1 litre (1¾ pints) of water, salt and pepper to taste, bring to the boil, and skim it. Simmer the stock for 20 minutes, strain and allow to cool. Skim again.

Sprinkle the gelatine over the stock and add the egg whites, beaten to stiff peaks, and the eggshells, crushed. (Do not stir them in.) Bring to the boil, stirring constantly, remove from the heat, and let stand for 20 minutes. Strain through a fine sieve lined with dampened kitchen towel, allow to cool and reserve 1 cup to coat the salmon. Chill the remainder until it has solidified. **Serves 3.**   **Carbohydrate: 2 grams.**

Braised Trout

2 trout	1 tbsp cider vinegar
½ cup white wine	¼ tsp ginger.

Grill or fry the fish until brown and then simmer in a dish with the other ingredients until the fish flakes easily. Place on a warm serving dish, reduce the cooking liquid by half, pour over the fish and serve. **Serves 2**   **Carbohydrate: 0**

Creole Prawns

4 slices bacon

1 medium chopped onion

25 g (1 oz) chopped green pepper

400 g (14 oz) tinned Italian tomatoes, drained, reserving ½ cup of juice, and chopped

300 ml (½ pint) chicken stock

12 leaves of Chinese cabbage

lard

25 g (1 oz) chopped celery

1 rounded tsp plain flour

100 g (4 oz) tomato juice

1 bay leaf

¼ tsp cayenne pepper

750 g (1½ lbs) prawns

Using a little lard, cook the bacon over a moderate heat in a large saucepan until it is crisp, then remove and crumble.

In the remaining fat, and on a low heat, cook the onion, celery and pepper until they are softened, add the flour and cook for a further 3 minutes. Add the tomatoes, reserved juice, tomato juice, bay leaf, broth and cayenne, bring to the boil and simmer for about 30 minutes, stirring, or until the sauce reaches the required consistency. Add the prawns, salt and pepper to taste, and simmer, stirring, for 3 or 4 minutes until the prawns are just cooked.

In the meantime, cut out the centre ribs of the Chinese leaves and chop them. Arrange the leaves, three to a plate, with the chopped ribs in the centre.

Pour the Creole prawns over the leaves and sprinkle it with the bacon.

Serves 3.   **Carbohydrate: 10 grams.**

Prawn Stuffed Courgettes

4 medium-sized courgettes (approx 100 g each)

lard

225 g (8 oz) prawns

2 tbsp lemon juice plus slices of lemon for garnish

black pepper

Put the courgettes into boiling salted water and cook for 10 minutes. Remove and drain. Using a little lard, sauté the prawns over a moderate heat. Slice the courgettes lengthwise. Pile the prawns on the courgettes and season with lemon juice and black pepper. Garnish with slices of lemon.

Serves 2.   **Carbohydrate: 10 grams.**

Poultry dishes

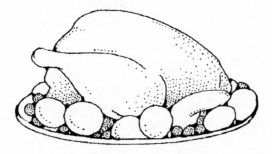

Chicken and Avocado Salad

½ head of romaine, rinsed, dried and chopped fine

½ iceberg lettuce, rinsed, dried and chopped fine

Small bunch curly endive rinsed, dried and chopped fine

½ bunch of watercress, coarse stems discarded, rinsed, dried and chopped fine

6 slices of bacon chopped fine

3 ripe avocados

2 chicken breasts (700 g, 1½ lbs) cooked and diced fine

1 tomato, chopped fine

1 hard-boiled egg separated, the yolk grated fine, the white grated fine

2 tbsp chopped fresh chives

1 tbsp red wine vinegar

2 tsp Dijon mustard

½ cup olive oil

50 g (2 oz) grated Cheddar cheese

In a large salad bowl, toss together the romaine, lettuce, endive and watercress. In a frying pan, fry the bacon over a moderate heat until it is crisp and remove it with a slotted spoon. Halve, pit and peel the avocados and cut into 15 mm (½ inch) pieces. Arrange the chicken, bacon, tomato and avocado decoratively over the greens and garnish with the grated egg and the chives.

In a small bowl, whisk together the vinegar, mustard, and salt and pepper to taste. Add the olive oil in a slow stream, whisking, and continue whisking until it is emulsified. Stir in the cheese. Whisk the dressing and pour over the salad.

Serves 6   **Carbohydrate: 7 grams.**

A low-carbohydrate stuffing recipe for chicken is included on page 136

Teriyake Chicken

2 tbsp soy sauce
½ tsp minced fresh ginger
5 tsp honey
1 tbsp medium Sherry

1 tbsp white wine vinegar
1 garlic clove, crushed with ½ tsp salt
450 g (1 lb) boneless chicken breast

In a bowl whisk together the soy sauce, ginger, honey, Sherry, vinegar and garlic paste. Flatten the chicken breasts between plastic wrap until they are about 15 mm (½ inch) thick. Marinate in the soy mixture for 20 minutes.

Transfer the chicken to a grill rack, skin sides down, reserving the marinade, and grill under a pre-heated grill, about 5 inches from the heat, for 5 minutes. While the chicken is cooking, boil the marinade until it is reduced by half. Brush the chicken with some of the marinade, turn it and brush with the remaining marinade. Grill the chicken until it is cooked through (about 7 minutes), transfer to a cutting board and cut it diagonally into 15 mm (½ inch) thick slices.

Serves 2.   **Carbohydrate: 8 grams.**

Chicken Galantine

A 2 kg (5 lb) chicken
120 g (4 oz) ground pork
25 g (1 oz) butter
120 g (4 oz) dried figs, chopped

1 tsp ground ginger
2 tsp cinnamon
1 tsp salt
pepper to taste

Loosen the skin at the chicken's breast. Cut the breasts out and chop small. Sauté the pork in butter until it is tender. Combine the chicken breasts, pork, figs, cinnamon, salt and pepper, and stuff the breast cavities under the skin. Skewer or sew to secure. Rub the chicken with butter and sprinkle with salt and pepper to taste. Roast in an oven at 180°C/350°F/Gas Mark 4 for 2½ hours basting frequently with butter.

May be served either hot or cold.

Serves 4-6.   **Carbohydrate: 7-5 grams**

Chicken with Herb Sauce

½ cup packed fresh parsley leaves
½ cup packed fresh tarragon leaves
2 sour gherkins, drained
2 small shallots, sliced thinly
4 whole chicken breasts (about 250 g, ½ lb each)

25 g (1 oz) butter
1 tbsp plain flour
½ cup chicken broth
½ cup double cream
1 tbsp Dijon mustard

In a food processor, chop fine the tarragon, parsley, gherkins and shallots. In a frying pan, fry the chicken in half the butter over a moderately high heat until it is browned lightly on both sides. Transfer to a plate and pour off the fat from the frying pan. Put the rest of the butter and the flour in the frying pan, return to the heat and cook the roux over a low heat for 3 minutes. Whisk in the broth and cook the mixture, whisking, until it has thickened. Stir in the cream, the parsley mixture and the mustard, add the chicken and cook it over a moderate heat until it is cooked through (about 5-6 minutes each side). Serve the chicken covered with the sauce.

Serves 4.   **Carbohydrate: 2 grams.**

Chicken with Cream and Currants

25 g (1 oz) clarified butter
4 boneless chicken breasts flattened between sheets of plastic wrap to about 4 mm (¼ inch)
4 small Granny Smith apples,

peeled, cored and sliced
1 tbsp dried currants
2 tsp crumbled, dried tarragon
2 tbsp Calvados
1 pint double cream

In a frying pan, heat the butter over a moderately high heat until it is hot but not smoking and sauté the chicken breasts in it until they are cooked through (4-5 minutes each side). Transfer the chicken to a plate and keep warm. Pour off all but 1 tablespoon of the fat from the frying pan, and in the remaining fat, sauté the apples, currants and tarragon over a low heat, stirring, until the apples are just tender. In a small saucepan, heat the Calvados until it is hot, ignite it, and pour it with care very slowly over the apple mixture. Cook the mixture until the flames subside and boil it until the liquid has thickened. Add the cream and salt and pepper to taste, pour it over the chicken.

Serves 4.   **Carbohydrate: 5 grams.**

Duck Breast with Chambord Sauce

4 boneless duck breasts about
   170g (6 oz) each
2 tbsp rendered duck fat (from
   making duck crackling, see
   below)
2 tsp sugar
4 tbsp red wine vinegar

6 tbsp dry red wine
2 tsp cornflour
225 ml (8 fl oz) chicken stock
3 tbsp Chambord (black raspberry
   flavoured liqueur)
25 g (1 oz) butter

Duck cracklings:
remove the skin from the duck breasts and chop. Lie the skin in a frying pan, just cover with water, bring to the boil and boil slowly, stirring occasionally, until the water has evaporated and the fat is rendered. Continue to cook the skin cracklings in the rendered fat at moderate heat, stirring, until they are golden. With a slotted spoon, transfer the cracklings to paper towels to drain and sprinkle with salt to taste. transfer the fat to a bowl to keep. The cracklings will keep for a week, the fat, indefinitely.

In a large frying pan heat 2 tablespoons of rendered duck fat over a moderate heat until it is hot but not smoking, and in it sauté the duck breasts, seasoned with salt and pepper, turning once, for 6 to 8 minutes or until they are just springy to the touch. Transfer to a cutting board and allow to stand for 5 minutes.

While the duck is standing, pour off the fat from the frying pan, add the sugar and vinegar and boil, stirring occasionally, until it is reduced to a glaze. Add the wine and boil until the mixture is reduced by half. Mix the cornflour in the stock and, stirring, add to the mixture in the frying pan with the Chambord. Bring to the boil, stirring and boil for 1 minute, remove from the heat, whisk in the butter until it is melted and incorporated and salt to taste. Spoon some onto four heated dinner plates, reserving the rest in a gravy boat. Slice the duck breasts thinly and arrange on the plates.

Serves 4.   **Carbohydrate: 4 grams.**

Turkey with Balsamic Vinegar and Honey Glaze

3 tbsp balsamic vinegar

1½ tsp honey

350 g (12 oz) turkey cutlets, about
   6 mm (¼ inch) thick

75 g (3 oz) bread crumbs seasoned
   with salt and pepper

25 g (1 oz) lard

3 garlic coves, crushed

15 g (½ oz) butter

120 ml (4 fl oz) dry white wine

chopped fresh parsley leaves for
   garnish

In a small bowl, mix the honey in the vinegar until it is dissolved. Dredge the
turkey in the breadcrumbs, pressing so that they adhere. In a large frying pan,
heat the lard over a moderately high heat until it is hot but not smoking, and
sauté the turkey in it, in batches, turning once, for 1 minute. Transfer to a
plate. Wipe out the frying pan, and cook the garlic in the butter, over a
moderately low heat, stirring, until it is golden (about 1 minute). stir in the
wine. Boil the mixture until the liquid is reduced to about 2 tablespoons, stir
in the vinegar and honey mixture, and boil until the mixture is syrupy. Spoon
the glaze over the turkey cutlets and sprinkle with parsley.

Serves 2.   **Carbohydrate: 7 grams.**

Turkey Blanquette

The following dish is useful if you have small pieces of turkey to use up.

225 g (8 oz) cold turkey, boned

40 g (1½ oz) butter

25 g (1 oz) flour

900 ml (¾ pint) light stock

pepper and salt to taste

a pinch of mace

1 egg yolk

2 tbsp cream

Cut the turkey into small pieces. In a saucepan, make a sauce with the butter,
flour and stock and cook it thoroughly. Season with the salt, pepper and mace
and remove from the heat. Add the egg yolk and cream and mix in quickly.
Reheat the turkey in the mixture without allowing it to boil. Serve with a
suitable garnish of rolls of bacon, grilled tomatoes or meatballs.

Serves 2.   **Carbohydrate: 12 grams**

Poultry is usually stuffed and the stuffing in most cases is largely carbohydrate. Below is a recipe for a chicken stuffing which dates back to the fifteenth century.

Roast Chicken Stuffing
for a 2½ kg (5 lb) chicken

12 hard-boiled egg yolks
200 g (8 oz) parsley, blanched and
chopped finely
110 g (4 oz) butter

¼ tsp ground ginger
½ tsp pepper
1 tsp salt
¼ tsp saffron (optional)

Hard-boil the eggs, halve and remove the yolks. Mix together all the ingredients and stuff the chicken.

Carbohydrate: 0

The egg whites may be saved and used as shells, stuffed with tuna fish, for example, in salads.

Meat dishes

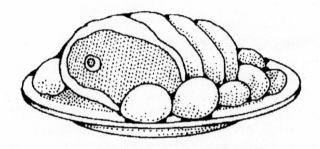

Roast beef with Salt Crust

1 cup coarse salt   1½-1¾ kg (3½-4 lbs) beef rib

In a bowl mix the salt with a little water until the mixture forms a slightly stiff paste resembling wet snow. Place the beef in a roasting pan, fat side up and coat it with the salt paste to about 6 mm (¼ inch) thick. Roast in a preheated oven at 160°C/325°F/Gas Mark 3, allowing 45 minutes per kg (22 minutes per pound) for medium-rare meat. Transfer to a cutting board, allow to stand for 15 minutes, break off the crust with a hammer and carve.

Serves 3-4.   **Carbohydrate: 0**

Meat Loaf with Almonds

Sauce   50 g (2 oz) fresh breadcrumbs
150 ml (¼ pint) cream or milk   4 tbsp red wine
20 g (¾ oz) coarsely ground almonds   1 tsp sugar
⅛ tsp bitter almond essence   ¼ tsp black pepper
                                         ⅛ tsp ground mace
900 g (2 lbs) ground beef   ⅛ tsp ground cloves

For the sauce. Simmer the cream, almonds and essence together for 10 minutes and allow to cool.

Combine all the ingredients in a bowl and shape to a loaf. Bake in a casserole at 160°C/325°F/Gas Mark 3, for 1 hour. Drain off the fat, turn out onto a serving plate and serve.

Serves 4-6.   **Carbohydrate: 1 gram**

Beef Steak in Pepper and Macadamia Nut Sauce

For the beef:

650 g (1½ lbs) beef steak cut into 4
1 tsp Worcestershire sauce
5 garlic cloves; 2 peeled and crus-
    hed, 3 left whole and unpeeled.
25 g (1 oz) butter
1 fresh sprig of thyme
1 fresh sprig of oregano

For the sauce:

1 sweet red pepper
1 tbsp beef broth
1 tbsp brandy
1 tbsp sour cream
15 g (½ oz) butter
1 tbsp chopped macadamia nuts

Beef: Rub the beef all over with the Worcestershire sauce, the minced garlic cloves and salt and pepper to taste. Let it marinate overnight in a covered glass dish. In a frying pan, just large enough to hold the beef, heat the butter with the thyme, oregano and the unpeeled garlic cloves, on a moderate heat until it is hot. In it cook the beef, turning it to brown on all sides, until it is cooked as required. Transfer the beef to a plate and keep warm, covered. Discard the thyme, oregano and garlic, but reserve the fat in the frying pan

The sauce: In a saucepan mix the pepper and broth and simmer until the peppers are tender (about 15 minutes). Purée in a blender until it is smooth. Add the purée and the brandy to the fat in the frying pan and boil, stirring, for 5 minutes. Whisk in the sour cream and cook over a moderate heat, whisking, until it is hot but not boiling, whisk in the butter a little at a time, whisking until it is incorporated and stir in the macadamia nuts. Add salt and pepper to taste. Slice the beef and serve with the sauce.

Serves 4.   **Carbohydrate: 2 grams.**

Caribbean Beef Pot Roast

30 g (1 oz) lard
4 pieces beef braising steak, about
    250 g (½ lbs) each

3 tbsp rum
2 tbsp tomato paste
8 pimiento-stuffed olives, chopped

In a frying pan heat the lard until it is hot but not smoking and brown the steak in it on all sides. Pour the fat from the pan and add the rum. Simmer the meat for 20 minutes, covered, stir in the tomato paste and salt and pepper to taste, and continue to simmer, covered, for a further 2 hours, basting occasionally. remove to serving plates. Skim the fat off the juices in the frying pan and stir in the olives. Reheat if necessary and spoon the sauce over the meat.

Serves 4.   **Carbohydrate: 1 gram.**

Beef Goulash

60 g (2 oz) fat bacon
lard
1 large onion, sliced finely
1 clove garlic, crushed
450 g (1 lb) stewing steak, cubed

1 tbsp plain flour
1 glass red wine
150 ml (5 fl oz) beef stock
1 bouquet garni
salt, pepper and paprika

Chop the bacon coarsely. In a medium-sized saucepan, heat the lard over a moderately high heat. Add the bacon, onion and garlic and sauté until they are softened but not brown (about 5 mins). Dredge the beef cubes in the flour and add to the bacon mixture. Stir vigorously until it is browned all over. Add the wine, the stock and the bouquet garni. Season liberally with salt, pepper and paprika. Simmer gently for 1-1½ hours. Remove the bouquet garni and serve.
Serves 3.   **Carbohydrate: 5 grams.**

American Meat Loaf

2 onions, peeled and chopped finely
3 tbsp celery, chopped finely
2 garlic cloves, crushed
1½ tsp dried thyme, crumbled
30 g (1 oz) butter
2 tsp salt
1½ tsp pepper
100 g (4 oz) mushrooms, chopped
    finely
680 g (1½ lbs) minced beef

350 g (12 oz) minced pork
100 g (4 oz) bread crumbs
2 large eggs beaten lightly
4 tbsp bottled chili sauce or ketchup
420 g tin of tomatoes, drained and
    chopped
3 tbsp fresh parsley, chopped finely
3 slices streaky bacon, halved
    crosswise

In a frying pan, cook the onion, celery, garlic and thyme in the butter over a moderately low heat, stirring, until the onion is soft. Add the salt, pepper and mushrooms and cook the mixture over a moderate heat, stirring, until the mushrooms are tender and the juice they have given off has evaporated (5 to 10 minutes). Transfer the mixture to a large bowl and allow to cool. To the bowl add the minced meats, eggs, half the chili, tomatoes and parsley and stir until it is mixed well. Form the mixture into a 175 mm by 250 mm (7 inch by 10 inch) loaf on a shallow baking tin, spread the remaining chili sauce over it and drape the bacon over the loaf. Bake the meat loaf in the middle of a pre-heated oven at 180°C/350°F/Gas Mark 4, for 1 hour.
Serves 6 to 8.   **Carbohydrate: 9 grams.**

Lamb Chops in Lemon Caper Sauce

Two 40 mm (1½ inch) thick lamb   1 tsp grated lemon zest
  chops or 4 smaller ones   1 tsp bottled capers, drained
15 g (½ oz) butter   1 tbsp lemon juice

Sprinkle the lamb chops with salt and pepper to taste and grill them under a pre-heated grill, about 100 mm (4 inches) from the heat for 6 minutes (less for the smaller chops). Turn over and grill for a further 4 minutes for medium rare meat. Let them stand for 5 minutes.

While the chops are standing, in a small saucepan, melt the butter and stir in the zest, the capers, lemon juice and salt and pepper to taste.

Transfer the chops to plates and pour the sauce over them.

Serves 2.   **Carbohydrate: negligible**

Herbed Roast Leg of Lamb with Onions

60 g (2 oz) Dijon mustard   75 ml (2 fl oz) dry white wine
1 large garlic clove crushed to a   2 tbsp olive oil
  paste with ¼ tsp salt   3.5 kg (8 lb) leg of lamb, pelvic
½ tbsp finely chopped fresh rose-   bone removed and tied
  mary or 1 tsp dried, crumbled   1 kg (2 lbs) small onions, blanched
  plus a fresh sprig for garnish   in boiling water for 2 minutes,
½ tbsp finely chopped fresh thyme   drained and peeled
  or 1 tsp dried, crumbled plus a   2 large carrots cut into 12 mm (½-
  fresh sprig for garnish   inch) pieces
1 tbsp soy sauce

Gravy   30 g (1 oz) butter, softened
1 cup red wine   2 tbsp plain flour
2 cups beef broth

In a small bowl whisk together the mustard, garlic, rosemary, thyme, soy sauce, and wine, adding salt and pepper to taste. Add 1 tablespoon of olive oil in a stream, whisking, and continue whisking until the mixture is thoroughly combined. Brush the lamb generously on all sides with some of the mixture, reserving the rest, and let it marinate in a lightly larded roasting pan, covered and chilled, for at least 6 hours and preferably overnight.

Let the lamb return to room temperature and brush it with the rest of the mustard mixture. In a bowl toss the onions in the rest of the oil, add them and the carrots to the baking pan and roast them with the lamb in the middle of a pre-heated oven at 230°C/450°F/Gas Mark 8 for 15 minutes. Reduce the temperature to 180°C/350°F/Gas Mark 4 and roast, stirring the vegetables occasionally, for 1 hour 15 minutes, for medium-rare meat. Transfer the lamb to a platter and let stand for 20 minutes. Transfer the onions with a slotted spoon to a serving dish, leaving the carrots in the pan, and keep them warm, covered.

To make the gravy: Pour off the fat from the pan, reserving the other juices. Transfer the juices and carrots to a saucepan and add the wine. Boil the mixture until it is reduced by half and mash the carrots. Add the broth and bring to the boil. In a small bowl knead together the butter and flour until they are combined well and add to the mixture a little at a time, whisking. Add salt and pepper and salt to taste. Simmer the gravy, whisking occasionally, until it is thickened (about 3 minutes).

Garnish the lamb with thyme and rosemary sprigs.

Serves 8.   **Carbohydrate: 2 grams.**

Lamb Chops with Mint Vinegar Sauce

Sauce:
2 tbsp white wine vinegar
2 tbsp granulated sugar
2 tbsp fresh spearmint leaves, minced

12 small lamb chops
1 garlic clove, halved across
½ tsp dried thyme, crumbled
white pepper to taste

For the sauce: In a small saucepan mix the vinegar and sugar and cook over a moderate heat, stirring, until the sugar has dissolved. Stir in the spearmint and let the mixture cool. Season the sauce with salt and pepper to taste and transfer to a bowl

Rub the chops with the cut sides of the garlic, and sprinkle them on both sides with the thyme and pepper. sauté in a larded pan over a moderately high heat, on both sides for about 2 minutes, for medium rare meat. Serve with the sauce.

Serves 4 or 6.   **Carbohydrate: 8 or 6 grams.**

Lamb Satay

1 medium onion, minced
1 garlic clove, crushed
1 tsp fresh coriander, chopped
1 tsp fresh ginger, minced and
    peeled
1 tbsp rice wine vinegar
1 tbsp vegetable oil
1 tsp Chinese chili paste
900 g (2 lbs) lamb shoulder cut
    into 20 mm (¾ inch) cubes
10 260 mm (10 inch) wooden
    skewers soaked in cold water
    for 30 minutes.

Sauce
12 g (½ oz) butter
25 g (1 oz) dry-roasted peanuts,
    crushed
3 shallots, chopped
1 garlic clove, crushed
½ tsp shrimp paste
½ tsp Chinese chili paste
1 tbsp fresh lemon juice

In a shallow dish, mix the onion, garlic, coriander, ginger, oil vinegar and chili. Add the lamb cubes, stirring to coat them with the marinade and let them marinate, covered, overnight.

Sauce: In a saucepan heat the butter until it is hot and in it cook the peanuts, shallots, garlic and shrimp paste, stirring, for 1 minute or until it has thickened. Add the chili paste and lemon juice and 1½ cups of water, and simmer for 5-7 minutes, or until it has thickened, stirring occasionally. Season with salt and pepper to taste.

Thread the lamb onto the skewers, grill for 10 minutes on each side and transfer to a serving plate. Pour the sauce over the lamb. Makes about 10 satays.

Serves 4-5.   **Carbohydrate: 5 grams.**

Pork and Bitter Orange

900 g (2 lbs) boneless loin of pork
    cut into 40 mm (1½ inch) pieces
140 ml (¾ cup) Seville orange juice,
    or 100 ml (½ cup) orange plus
    40 ml (¼ cup) lemon juice
1 tsp dried oregano, crumbled

1 tsp ground cumin
1 tsp ground white pepper
10 garlic cloves
1 bay leaf
1 large Spanish onion, chopped

In an ovenproof casserole mix the pork with the orange juice, oregano, cumin, pepper, garlic, bay leaf and onion and let it marinate, covered, for at least 3 hours or overnight, stirring occasionally. Bake the pork mixture, covered, in the middle of a pre-heated oven at 160°C/325°F/Gas Mark 3, until the pork is tender(about 3 to 3½ hours), discard the bay leaf and serve the pork mixture with mixed vegetables.

Serves 4 to 6.   **Carbohydrate: 1 gram** (plus vegetables)

Baked Ham with Mushroom, Cucumber and Tarragon Sauce

15 g (½ oz) butter
4 large mushrooms, sliced thinly
½ cucumber, peeled, seeded and sliced thinly, across
2 tsp fresh chopped tarragon leaves
plus sprigs for garnish
2 tbsp double cream
¼ tsp Dijon mustard
350 g (12 oz) ham steak

In a frying pan, melt the butter over a moderate heat until the foam subsides and in it cook the mushrooms, stirring, until they begin to give off their liquid. Add the cucumber and cook the mixture, stirring, until the cucumber is softened slightly (about 3-5 minutes). Stir in the chopped tarragon, cream and mustard and cook until the mixture has thickened slightly.

Put the ham in a baking dish and cover with the mushroom mixture. Bake the ham in the middle of a pre-heated oven at 180°C/350°F/Gas Mark 4, for 10 minutes, or until it is heated through. Serve garnished with tarragon sprigs.

Serves 2.   **Carbohydrate: 7 grams.**

Microwaved Pork Chops with Peppers

1 tsp butter
two 25 mm (1 inch) thick pork chops
2 tbsp chicken stock
2 tbsp plus 1 tsp balsamic vinegar
1 sweet red pepper, chopped coarsely
1 sweet green pepper, chopped
1 tsp cornstarch dissolved in 2 tsp water.

In a frying pan, heat the butter over a moderately high heat until the foam has subsided, and in it brown the chops which have been seasoned with salt and pepper. Add the stock and vinegar and bring to the boil. Transfer to a microwave-safe baking dish, just large enough for the chops in one layer, sprinkle with the sweet peppers. Cover with microwave-safe plastic wrap and cook at medium power (50%) for 6 minutes. Stir the cornstarch mixture into

the cooking juices and microwave the mixture, covered, at high power (100%) for 1 minute.
Serves 2.   **Carbohydrate: 5 grams.**

Roast Peppercorn Pork

2 kg (4½ lb) pork loin boned and
  rolled
40 g (1½ oz) butter, softened
2 tbsp plain flour
2 tbsp mixed white, black, green and
  pink peppercorns, crushed coarse

Gravy:
2 tbsp plain flour
350 ml (12 fl oz) chicken stock
2 tbsp red wine vinegar

Season the pork with salt. In a bowl mix the butter and flour to a paste, coat the top of the pork with it and sprinkle the peppercorns on the paste. Press them slightly so that they stick. Roast the pork in the middle of a pre-heated oven at 240°C/475°F/Gas Mark 9 for 30 minutes, reduce the heat to 160°C/325°F/Gas Mark 3 and roast until the pork is cooked through (about a further 1 hr 30 mins). Transfer to a cutting board and let stand for 10 minutes.

Gravy: Pour off the fat from the roasting pan reserving 2 tablespoons, whisk in the flour and cook over a moderate heat, stirring, for 3 minutes. Add the stock and about 1 cup of water from cooking green vegetables or plain water, in a stream, whisking, and bring to the boil. Stir in the vinegar and salt and pepper to taste. Simmer until is has thickened as desired. Transfer to a gravy boat.

Carve the pork into 15 mm (½ inch) slices.
Serves 8-10.   **Carbohydrate: 2 grams.**

Egg and Cheese (Vegetarian) dishes

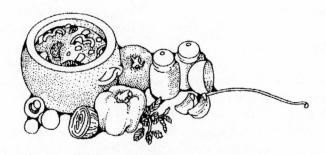

Goat Cheese and Walnut Soufflé

75 g (3 oz) walnuts, toasted lightly, cooled and finely chopped.
30 g (1 oz) unsalted butter
1½ tbsp plain flour
150 ml (4 fl oz) milk

2 large eggs, separated.
75 g (3 oz) grated mild goat's cheese
¼ tsp crumbled dry thyme leaves
cream of tartar, a pinch.

Butter 4 half-cup ramekins, coat the bottom and sides of each with about 1 tsp of walnuts and place the ramekins on a baking tray.

In a small saucepan, melt the butter over a low heat, mix in the flour and cook, whisking, for 3 minutes. Add the milk in a stream, whisking, and boil over a moderate heat, whisking, until the mixture is thick and smooth (about 2 minutes). Transfer the mixture to a bowl to cool slightly. Whisk in the egg yolks, one at a time, the cheese and thyme, and salt and pepper to taste. Mix well.

In another bowl, beat the egg whites with a pinch of salt until they are frothy, add the cream of tartar. Beat until the whites maintain stiff peaks. Whisk one third of the whites into the cheese mixture and fold in the rest gently but thoroughly. Divide the soufflé mixture between the ramekins, sprinkle the remaining walnuts equally on each soufflé and bake in the top of a pre-heated oven at 200°C/400°F/Gas Mark 6 for 20 minutes, or until they are puffed and golden.

Serves 4.   **Carbohydrate content: 10 grams.**

Serve with chicory and watercress salad.

Cheese and Tomato Soufflés

25 g (1 oz) butter

1 tbsp plain flour

¼ l (½ pint) milk

2 tbsp tomato paste

1 cup grated Swiss cheese

2 tbsp grated Parmesan cheese

cayenne pepper to taste

3 large eggs, separated

1 tbsp medium sherry

In a saucepan melt the butter over a low heat, stir in the flour and cook the roux, stirring, for 3 minutes. Bring the milk to the boil. Remove the roux pan from the heat and add the scalded milk, in a stream, whisking vigorously until the mixture is thick and smooth. Simmer the sauce for 3-4 minutes, or until it has thickened, and whisk in the tomato paste, cheeses, cayenne and salt to taste. Continue whisking until the cheeses have melted. Remove from the heat and whisk in the egg yolks, one at a time, beating each well in. Transfer to a bowl to cool.

In a bowl, whisk the egg whites with a pinch of salt, until they maintain soft peaks, add the Sherry and beat the mixture until it maintains stiff peaks. Fold the egg-white mixture into the cheese mixture gently but thoroughly, transfer to 6 buttered ramekins, and bake the soufflés in the middle of a preheated oven at 200°C/400°F/Gas Mark 6 for 25-30 minutes, or until they are cooked through.

Serves 6.   **Carbohydrate: 4 grams.**

Blue Cheese Omelette

60 g (2 oz) blue cheese, crumbled

2 tbsp double cream

4 large eggs

¼ tsp salt

¼ tsp pepper

25 g (1 oz) butter

In a bowl stir together the cheese and the cream. In another bowl, beat the eggs with a fork and stir in the salt and pepper. In a frying pan, heat the butter over a moderate heat until the foam begins to subside, add the egg mixture and cook it, covered.

When the top begins to firm, spoon the cheese mixture over the omelette and cook until the cheese mixture thickens (about 2 minutes). Fold the omelette in half over the cheese filling and serve.

Serves 2.   **Carbohydrate: 0**

Savoury Cheesecake

2 tbsp grated Parmesan
2 tbsp fine dry bread crumbs
425 ml (¾ pint) double cream
250 g (8 oz) blue cheese, crumbled

680 g (1½ lbs) cream cheese, cut
   into pieces and softened
4 large eggs

In a bowl mix well the Parmesan and breadcrumbs and coat the inside of a 9 inch cake tin. In a saucepan scald the cream. In a large bowl, with an electric whisk, blend the blue cheese with 2 tablespoons of the cream until the mixture is smooth, add half the cream cheese and beat until it is smooth. Beat in the remaining cream and beat until it is smooth. add the remaining cream cheese and beat until it is smooth. Beat in the eggs, one at a time, and beat until the mixture is smooth. Pour the mixture into the prepared cake tin. Bake the cheesecake in the bottom of a preheated oven at 160°C/325°F/Gas Mark 3, until the centre is just firm (about 1 hr 15 minutes).

Let the cheesecake cool completely, preferably overnight. Turn the cheesecake out and serve sliced thinly.

Serves 6-8.   **Carbohydrate: negligible**

Baked Stuffed Eggs

60 g (2 oz) butter
2 shallots, minced
6 mushrooms, chopped finely
2 tbsp milk
2 tbsp single cream
2 tbsp dry white wine
6 large hard-boiled eggs

Sauce:
25 g (1 oz) butter
2 tbsp plain flour
430 ml (¾ pint) milk, scalded
140 g (5 oz) Gruyère cheese, grated
1 egg yolk

In a frying pan heat the butter until it is hot and sauté the shallots over a moderate heat, stirring occasionally, until they are softened (about 4 minutes). Add the mushrooms, milk, cream and wine, and simmer the mixture, stirring occasionally, for 15 minutes. Allow to cool.

Halve the eggs lengthwise, remove the yolks and crumble them in a bowl. Stir in the mushroom mixture and combine well. Add salt and pepper to taste. Divide the mixture between the egg whites, place one half on top of another and reform each egg into its original shape.

Sauce: In a saucepan melt the butter over a low heat, stir in the flour and cook over a moderate heat, stirring for 3 minutes. Remove from the heat and add the scalded milk in a stream, whisking, and cook the mixture, whisking vigorously, until it is smooth and has thickened. Remove from the heat and stir in half the Gruyère, egg yolk and salt and pepper to taste. Spoon one third of the sauce to an oven-proof serving dish, just large enough to hold the eggs, cover them with the remaining sauce, sprinkle with the remaining half of the Gruyère, and bake them in the upper third of a pre-heated very hot oven at 260°C/500°F/Gas Mark 10, until the cheese is bubbly and browned slightly (about 10 minutes).

Serves 6.   **Carbohydrate: 7 grams.**

Eggs with Anchovies

12 eggs   4 anchovies, crushed
85 g (3 oz) butter   3-4 tbsp beef or lamb stock, or white
30 g (1 oz) pistachio nuts, shelled   wine
    and crushed   Iceberg lettuce leaves

Scramble the eggs in the butter over a low heat while stirring in the nuts. Purée the anchovies in the stock and stir into the eggs as they begin to harden. Serve on the lettuce leaves or with a salad.

Serves 6.   **Carbohydrate: negligible**

Salads

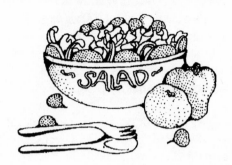

The following salads are not designed to eaten alone but as accompaniments to cold meats, fish, etc.

Mushroom Salad

3 tbsp olive oil
1½ tbsp plain yogurt
1½ tbsp lemon juice
3 tbsp sour cream
1 tsp minced shallot or onion
1 large garlic clove, crushed to a
pulp
½ tsp salt
2 tbsp minced fresh parsley
450 g (1 lb) button mushrooms
ground white pepper to taste.

Mix together the oil, yogurt, lemon juice, sour cream, shallot, garlic, salt and parsley in a bowl. Toss the mushrooms in the mixture gently but thoroughly. Season with salt and pepper to taste.
Serves 4-6.

Carbohydrate: 4 grams.

Chicory and Watercress Salad

1 tbsp sherry (or white wine) vinegar
½ tsp Dijon mustard
2 tbsp walnut oil
1 tbsp olive oil
1 large bunch watercress, rinsed,
dried and coarse, stems discarded
1 chicon of French or Italian chicory,
rinsed and dried.

Whisk together the vinegar, mustard. Add the oils in a stream, whisking, and add salt and pepper to taste. Whisk until emulsified. Toss the watercress and chicory in the dressing.
Serves 4.

Carbohydrate: 2 grams.

Blue Cheese and Walnut Winter Salad

1 small head of radicchio, separated, rinsed, dried and torn into small pieces

1 small head of lettuce, separated, rinsed, dried and torn into small pieces

1 bunch of watercress, rinsed dried and coarse stems discarded

1 endive, leaves separated and torn in half

Dressing:

3 shallots, peeled

2 tbsp white wine vinegar

½ tsp salt

¼ tsp pepper

½ cup extra-virgin olive oil

1 tsp walnut oil

36 walnut halves, toasted

250 g (½ lb) blue cheese, crumbled

Toss together the raddichio, lettuce, watercress and endive.

Make the dressing: Under a moderately high heat, grill the shallots on each side until they turn golden and are fragrant (about 5-6 minutes). Let them cool and chop fine. In a bowl, combine the shallots, vinegar, salt, and pepper, add the oils in a stream, whisking, and whisk until the dressing has emulsified.

Pour the dressing over the salad and add the walnuts and cheese. Toss to combine it well and serve.

Serves 4-6.   **Carbohydrate: 13 grams.**

Parmesan and Anchovy Salad

3 garlic cloves

3 anchovy fillets, drained and mashed

2 large egg yolks

2 tsp white-wine vinegar

2 tsp balsamic vinegar

1½ tsp Dijon mustard

1 tsp Worcestershire sauce

¼ tsp salt

1½ tsp lime juice

¾ cup extra-virgin olive oil

2 heads of romaine, rinsed, dried and torn into strips

40 g (1½ oz) Parmesan cheese, grated.

Crush the garlic and mash with the anchovies to form a paste. Whisk the paste with the egg yolks, vinegars, mustard, Worcestershire sauce, salt and lime juice. Add the oil in a stream and whisk until emulsified.

Toss the romaine and Parmesan in a bowl, add the dressing and toss until combined well.

Serves 4-6.   **Carbohydrate: 3 grams.**

Watercress and Radicchio Salad

1 tbsp white wine vinegar
½ tsp Dijon mustard
2 tsp fresh parsley leaves, chopped
1 tbsp extra-virgin olive oil
2 bunches watercress, washed, dried

and separated into sprigs
2 small heads of radicchio, washed, dried and shredded fine
3 spring onions, sliced
175 g (6 oz) Parmesan, grated

In a small bowl, whisk together the vinegar, parsley, and salt and pepper to taste. Add the oil in a stream, whisking the dressing until it has emulsified.

In a salad bowl, toss together the watercress, radicchio and spring onions. Pour the dressing over the salad and toss well. Cover with Parmesan.

Serves 8.   **Carbohydrate: 3 grams.**

Mushroom, Radish and Endive Salad

½ tsp Dijon mustard
1 tbsp red wine vinegar
2 tbsp extra-virgin olive oil
8 leaves of soft lettuce, rinsed and dried

4 radishes, trimmed and sliced thinly
4 button mushrooms, sliced thinly
1 large endive, trimmed and cut across into 6 mm (¼ inch) slices
sprig of fresh parsley leaves

In a salad bowl, whisk together the mustard, vinegar and salt to taste. Add the oil a little at a time, whisking and whisk the dressing until it has emulsified. Add the lettuce, radishes, mushrooms, endive, and parsley and pepper to taste, and toss the salad to coat.

Serves 2.   **Carbohydrate: 5 grams**

Salad dressings

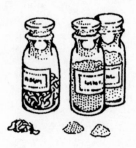

Mayonnaise

2 large egg yolks
2 tsp wine vinegar
1 tsp Dijon mustard, or to taste
¼ tsp salt
white pepper to taste

400 ml (12 fl oz) olive oil or
    vegetable oil
fresh lemon juice to taste
single cream to thin the mayonnaise
    as required

Warm a mixing bowl with hot water and dry well. In the bowl, combine the egg yolks, 1 teaspoon of vinegar, the mustard, salt and pepper. Beat or whisk vigorously until the mixture is well combined. Add ½ cup of oil, drop by drop, beating constantly. Add the remaining teaspoon of vinegar and the remaining cup of oil in a stream, whisking constantly. Add the lemon juice, white pepper and salt to taste and thin with cream as required.

Makes about 1 ltr.   **Carbohydrate: 0**

Cooked Mayonnaise

5 egg yolks
1 tbsp cornflour
2 tbsp extra-virgin olive oil

2 tbsp lemon juice
½ cup of hot water
ground white pepper to taste

In a small saucepan, combine the yolks with the cornflour, add the oil in a slow stream, whisking, and whisk in the lemon juice and the hot water. Cook over a moderately low heat, whisking constantly, until it thickens. Remove from the heat, season with salt and pepper to taste, and transfer to a jar. Chill the mayonnaise until it is cold.

Makes about 1 cup.   **Carbohydrate: 7 grams.**

Green Goddess Dressing

1 garlic clove halved
8 anchovy fillets, drained, reserving
   1 tsp of the oil
1 minced spring onion
1 tsp minced fresh tarragon leaves

½ tbsp minced fresh parsley leaves
2 tsp minced fresh chives
2 tsp tarragon vinegar
1 cup mayonnaise

Rub a bowl with the cut garlic. In the bowl, mash the anchovies with the reserved oil, add the spring onion, tarragon, parsley, chives and vinegar and mayonnaise. Combine well. (At this stage the mixture will be very thick. It may be thinned with water to the desired consistency.) The dressing may be used thick as a dip with prawns or vegetables, or thinned on salads or white fish.

Carbohydrate: negligible

Chili Dressing

1 tbsp double cream
3 tbsp mayonnaise
1 tbsp chili bottled sauce
2 tbsp finely chopped fresh parsley

1 small onion, finely chopped
1 tbsp finely chopped chives
⅛ tsp cayenne pepper

Whip the cream until it just maintains soft peaks. Whisk the other ingredients in a bowl. Fold in the whipped cream gently but thoroughly.

Carbohydrate: Negligible

Hard Egg Hollandaise

3 hard-boiled egg yolks
4 tsp lemon juice
100 g (4 oz) butter

finely chopped fresh herbs, if desired, to taste

Blend the yolks in a food processor until they are smooth, add 2 tablespoons of boiling water and the lemon juice and blend the mixture until it is smooth and fluffy. In a small saucepan, heat the butter over a moderate heat until it begins to foam. With the food processor running, pour in the butter slowly in a thin stream and season to taste with the herbs, salt and white pepper.

Makes about 1 cup.   **Carbohydrate: 1 gram.**

Saffron Garlic Mayonnaise

¼ tsp saffron threads   3 garlic cloves, crushed
2 tsp lemon juice   pinch of cayenne
285 ml (½ pint) mayonnaise

Put the saffron on a saucer, on a rack over a saucepan of boiling water and let the saffron steam until it is brittle (3 or 4 minutes). Remove and crumble the saffron into a bowl. In the bowl, whisk in the saffron, lemon juice, mayonnaise, garlic paste and cayenne until the mixture is well combined.

Serve with fish soups, grilled seafood or chicken.

Makes about half a cup.   **Carbohydrate: 1 gram.**

Desserts

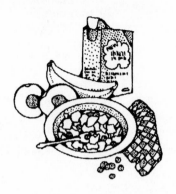

Baked Egg Custard

3 large eggs
600 ml (1 pint) full cream milk
½ tsp vanilla essence

6-8 drops liquid or granulated
   artificial sweetener
1 pinch of nutmeg

Break the eggs into an ovenproof dish and beat lightly. In a small saucepan, heat the milk but do not allow to boil. Add the sweetener and vanilla essence. Pour into the egg mixture while stirring to ensure it is well mixed. Sprinkle with nutmeg. Place the dish in a tray of water and bake in a cool oven (150°C/300°F/ Gas Mark 2) until the custard is just set (about 1 hour).
Serves 4.   **Carbohydrate: 8 grams.**

Apple Snow

450 g (1 lb) cooking apples
2 egg whites
juice and zest of 1 lemon

liquid or granulated artificial
   sweetener to taste

Make a shallow cut around the middle of each apple. Put in a baking dish and bake in a moderate oven (180°C/350°F/Gas Mark 4) for 30 minutes. Remove the pulp from the apples and press it through a sieve. Add sweetener to taste and leave the mixture to cool. Meanwhile beat the egg whites until stiff. Add the apple mixture a little at a time. Put in decorative dishes, chill well and serve.
Serves 4.   **Carbohydrate: 10 grams.**

Lemon Soufflé

4 large eggs, separated
juice and zest of 1 lemon
3 tbsp caster sugar

Beat the egg yolks with the lemon and sugar until the mixture is light and frothy. Whip the egg whites until stiff and fold into the lemon mixture. Pour into a buttered soufflé dish and bake in a hot oven (200°C/400°F/Gas Mark 6) for 10 minutes. This dish should be made as quickly as possible and served immediately.

Serves 4.   **Carbohydrate: 12 grams.**

Apple Fritters

75 g (3 oz) flour   3 apples
4 eggs   caster sugar for garnish
a pinch of pepper   450 g (1 lb) lard for frying
⅛ tsp saffron (optional)

Beat the eggs and mix with the flour to make a smooth batter. Add the pepper and saffron.

Peel, core and slice the apples, put them in the batter and leave for 1 hour to allow the saffron to colour and flavour the batter. Heat the lard in a deep pan until it begins to boil. Into it place large spoonfuls of the mixture and fry for about 3-4 minutes or until golden brown. Drain, sprinkle with sugar and serve hot.

Serves 3.   **Carbohydrate: 35 grams**

Wine Custard

4 whole eggs and two yolks   ½ tsp ground cloves
400 ml (1 pint) red wine   ½ tsp mace
50 g (2 oz) sugar   a pinch each of ginger, nutmeg and
½ tsp cinnamon   cinnamon

Beat the eggs in a bowl. Heat the wine and whisk it into the eggs. Stir in the sugar, cinnamon, cloves and mace. Stir over a low heat until it thickens. Pour into a serving dish and allow to cool. Sprinkle very lightly with ginger, nutmeg and cinnamon. Serve with baked apples or with vanilla ice-cream.

Serves 4.   **Carbohydrate: 20 grams.**

Real Vanilla Ice-cream

4 large eggs
100 g (4 oz) caster sugar

400 ml (½ pint) cream
vanilla essence

Separate the eggs. In a bowl, whisk the egg whites until they are stiff. Add the yolks and sugar.

In another bowl, whip the cream until it is stiff. Combine the cream and the egg mixture and add the vanilla essence, then freeze.

Serves 4.   **Carbohydrate: 25 grams**

Alternative ice-cream recipes

Some very nice ice-creams can be made quickly and easily using just cream and a sweetened flavour. For example: Using whipping cream, whip until it is stiff and combine with lemon curd, black cherry jam, or any other smooth jam.

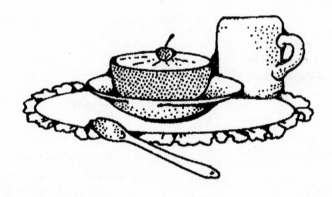

Recipe Index

About the Author

Barry Groves lives with his wife, Monica, in the Cotswold village of Milton under Wychwood. He trained as an electronic engineer and was commissioned in the Royal Air Force with which he served until 1982.

In 1962 he had developed a personal interest in the role of food types in the aetiology of obesity. When he retired from the RAF, at the age of 45, he took up full-time research into this and broadened the scope of his research to the relationship between diet and other modern diseases such as heart disease and cancers.

As a result of his researches, he realised that the perceived wisdoms, both of low-calorie dieting for weight loss and 'healthy eating' for the control of heart disease, were seriously flawed. The public were being misled largely, it seemed, to increase the profits of commercial interests.

He began to give talks and lectures, at first locally and then, increasingly over an ever-wider area. However, he realised that to reach more people a book was needed. In 1988 he bought a computer, taught himself to use it, and began to write.

In the 1980s, he served as a West Oxfordshire District Councillor. From 1987 to 1989 he was Chairman of the Public Health Committee.

Barry Groves does not confine himself to medical and dietary research. With a long-term interest in energy conservation, he and his wife, Monica, designed and built their own solar-heated house over three years from 1977 to 1980.

For relaxation, in 1982, he took up archery. With his compound bow, he became the British Clout Archery Champion in 1987 at his first attempt. He retained this championship in the subsequent four years, holding all the British Records in this discipline from 1989 to 1992. After silver medals in 1992 and 1993, he regained this championship in 1994.

In 1992 he entered the British Flight Archery Championships, winning with a British record. He has successfully defended this championship ever since with a further 5 British Records.

In 1996 he was invited to compete in the World Flight Archery Championships in California. Using a homemade bow, the world's first compound flight bow, he won all three of his classes with two World Records. In the 1997 World Championships in Nevada, he again took three Gold Medals with a further two World Records.